ARTHRITIS

By the same Author:
Allergies
Menopause
Stress

NUTRITIONAL HEALTH SERIES

ARTHRITIS

Stephen Terrass

Thorsons
An Imprint of HarperCollins*Publishers*

To Nicola, whose love, understanding, patience, encouragement and valuable input have helped me immeasurably in the writing of the book.

Thorsons
An Imprint of HarperCollins*Publishers*
77–85 Fulham Palace Road,
Hammersmith, London W6 8JB
1160 Battery Street,
San Francisco, California 94111–1213

Published by Thorsons 1994

10 9 8 7 6 5 4 3 2

A catalogue record for this book is available from the British Library

ISBN 0 7225 2983 X

Printed in Great Britain by HarperCollinsManufacturing, Glasgow

CONTENTS

ACKNOWLEDGEMENTS

The author wishes to thank the following for their valuable support and assistance in this project: Richard Passwater, Ph.D. for his inspiration, and for providing the Foreword and reviewing the manuscript; editor Sarah Sutton and copy-editor Barbara Vesey; special thanks to Rand Skolnick, John Steenson, Cheryl Thallon and Leyanne Scharff for their valuable support; and Nibs Laskor for his help and generosity. Most of all, fondest thanks to Nicola Squire and Shirley Terrass for their love and encouragement.

Arthritis is not a disease, but a group of diseases, commonly classed as either rheumatoid or osteoarthritis. It is believed that arthritis has been around for some time. Scientific literature tells us that the fossil of a large, swimming reptile called the platycarpus, which lived almost 100 million years ago, showed evidence of arthritis. Signs have also been detected in the bones of cavemen, and in the spines of several 8,000-year-old Egyptian mummies. And in Roman times, it was considered such a burden that the emperor Diocletian exempted citizens with severe arthritis from taxes.

In its various forms, arthritis is all too common. The author remarks that the most prevalent form, osteoarthritis, affects more than three out of four people over the age of 50. A fatalist would say that arthritis is almost a certainty – like death and taxes. As Stephen Terrass points out, however, this is far from the truth. In this book, which is relevant to *everyone*, he shows you how to prevent arthritis, as well as how to relieve the symptoms and even how to conquer the very disease process itself.

The first step is to realize that it is not a certainty that you suffer, but that diet and supplements can be the difference between health and arthritis. The anatomy of the disease is explained so that you can understand the condition and how diet is involved. The author's nutritional approach is proven, natural and has no adverse effects. He clearly instructs you in each step required to prevent arthritis, to treat symptoms without drugs, to correct many of the factors that cause or perpetuate the disease process, and to repair the damage. He also discusses conventional medical treatments and their limitations and risks.

This book shows you that there really is something you can do about arthritis. Death and taxes, however, are another matter.

Richard A. Passwater Ph.D.
February 1994

One could safely say that one of the ultimate visions of the average person in our society would be the obliteration of all health problems known to humanity. The fact that health, and consequently ill health, touch on all our lives makes us better understand this wish.

The problem is that although people take ill health so seriously, they do not often believe that they can play a part in eliminating it from their lives. People give millions to health charities each year in the hope that the money will help to put an end to a particular disease, and such donations *are* very valuable to the cause of research. The next step, of course, would be to utilize the results of the research that has already been undertaken. This is where the real tangible benefits of such research could be seen.

In the case of almost every health problem that plagues society today, research points very clearly to the fact that we, ourselves hold much of the ability to eliminate such problems. That is not to say that we do not need medicine nor those who carry out any necessary treatment; what it means is that the only guaranteed cure for most of these problems is *prevention*.

Unfortunately, very few people actually live their lives from a preventative point of view, presumably because, usually, only immediate concerns have any great bearing on our actions. From the perspective of health, however, this can be very damaging.

It must be said, though, that while this state of affairs may be our responsibility, it is mostly not our fault. After all, how often have you been taken by the hand and directed to a way of life that would help you to avoid a particular disease? The point is, if you do not know that there is something *you* can do about these problems, then no one can blame you for having them!

Fortunately for all of us, the necessary information is there for us to use and benefit from, if only we know where to look for it. That is not to say that, once given the information, we will use it. How many people have been told to stop smoking or lose weight in order to avoid a heart attack? And how many have taken this advice? Nevertheless, all of us should be given the opportunity to find such advice and then implement our findings if we so choose. It would be worth the effort if even one person was able to eliminate his or her suffering.

There are few better examples of the importance of this than in the case of arthritis. Without question, arthritis is among the most well known of all health disorders. Ironically, the fact that it is so well known has, in a way, perpetuated its ever more frequent occurrence. Most of us see arthritis as a very common but not life-threatening disorder, hence we are unduly casual about it. We all know many people who suffer with arthritis, and we are therefore more likely to assume that it is not preventable. This assumption is not only incorrect but is also the perfect example of a self-fulfilling prophecy. It is no secret that in Western society arthritis is getting, if anything, more common. Perhaps part of this is due to the fact that the typical 'Western' way of life includes certain factors that accentuate the risk of contracting arthritis, and the 'it is probably going to happen to me anyway' type of thinking means that the average person is unlikely to try to find out whether there really is something he or she can do about it.

The growing opinion states that because there is 'nothing one can do' about health problems such as arthritis, the best thing to do is to live life to the fullest while you can. On the surface this is a laudable approach, but it belies two very disturbing concerns. First, there *is* something that can be done about such problems; secondly, many of the factors involved in 'enjoying life to the fullest' – such as eating and/or drinking the wrong things and in excess – may well increase the risks.

Clearly, the most important first step is to realize that the risks of arthritis are quite high in our society today, but also that there are things that can be done; this refers not only to treating arthritis once it occurs, but to preventing most types of arthritis in the first place.

People have not been helped much in their understanding of arthritis by the rather generic use of the term. The limitations of this can be seen not only when it comes to identifying a person's *real* problem, but also in treating it. You see, although arthritis has a generic definition that is certainly medically appropriate, the fact that there are several different types of arthritis is often overlooked. No one has just 'arthritis'; sufferers have a particular form of arthritis, and unless they know what type they have, their efforts to treat it will be somewhat or even greatly impaired.

Once this is realized and a person is able to receive proper guidance, the way is paved either to reduce the risk of such problems significantly in the first place, or perhaps to relieve and/or reverse an already existing problem.

This book will take you through all the necessary steps to help you achieve such goals. First of all, it will help you to understand and recognize the various types of arthritis. Then it will give you a detailed explanation and practical guidelines to show you how arthritis symptoms and, in many cases, even the propensity to arthritis can either be treated or prevented. The guidelines discuss how various vitamins, minerals and herbs, and other natural agents can be combined with proper dietary management to formulate an effective 'anti-arthritis' programme. All the natural substances mentioned in these guidelines are medically and/or scientifically researched and very safe.

Whether you suffer from occasional nagging joint pain or a more serious arthritic disorder, it is important to understand your condition thoroughly and to strive to find answers to your problem. The information in this book should provide you with these answers and may help you to control your arthritis once and for all!

CHAPTER 1

What Is Arthritis?

In spite of the fact that arthritis is such a common and well-known health disorder, few people know a great deal about what the condition entails. There are also a great many misconceptions as to its actual definition.

Arthritis literally means 'inflammation of the joint'. As mentioned in the Introduction, the rather generic use of the term arthritis is not very helpful either in diagnosing the condition, or in treating it. While it is true that joint inflammation is a standard feature of any form of arthritis, this is not the condition's only characteristic by any means; as a matter of fact, sometimes it is not even the most important one!

All too often, treating a condition 'generically' that actually takes many different forms leads to the unfortunate mistake of addressing only its symptoms. Where arthritis is concerned, this is often taken to an extreme, so that only *one* symptom – that of the joint inflammation – is dealt with.

So what is so bad about this? Aren't sufferers only really concerned with eliminating the primary symptom nagging them so much?

It may well be that many sufferers would be satisfied if their main symptoms were relieved. One problem with this approach is that it can leave sufferers unaware of the fact that other methods can be used to alleviate their pain. Another problem stems from the fact that the standard treatments of the symptoms often have symptoms of their own, in the form of side-effects. Thirdly, suppressing the main symptom of an arthritic disorder does *not* treat the condition itself.

It is clear that if you intend to actually treat the *cause* as well as *all* the symptoms of the various kinds of arthritis, you need first to understand all the aspects of the form of arthritis you have. Only then can you achieve real control over your condition – over both its symptoms and its cause.

In order to give you the necessary background to the different types of arthritis, we need to look first at the basic mechanics of the joints.

THE JOINTS

'Joint' is a term used to refer to the meeting point between two or more bones in the body. There are actually different types of joints in the body. Each type of joint has particular characteristics that differentiate it from the others. Once equipped with a description of each type, you can begin to get a picture of how that joint works and, conversely, how the same type of joint can be damaged.

Many of the joints in your body are mobile, or allow for movement, while certain ones are immobile. The three primary classifications of joints are *synovial joints*, *cartilaginous joints* and *fibrous joints*.

Synovial Joints

Most joints in the body are synovial joints. They have varying degrees of mobility; in your shoulders, for instance, these joints allow for a vast range of movement, while certain joints in your hands allow for only a limited range. The bones that meet in synovial joints have semi-rounded ends. These semi-rounded ends are covered with a protective coating called *cartilage*. (Cartilage is a substance that will be referred to again and again in this book. As you will find, it is one of the most important factors in the subject of arthritis.) Cartilage contains large amounts of a substance called *collagen*. Collagen is a protein that acts as a sort of 'cement' for the cells of various tissues in the body. The apparent smoothness of the cartilage coating helps give the ends of the bones in a joint more 'friction-free' mobility, as well as helping to protect the bones from making contact with one another.

The cartilage, however, could not accomplish this on its own in a synovial joint. The actual bones in synovial joints are not really intended to connect with or touch one another; they are protected from this by the cartilage, a synovial membrane and synovia, and ligaments.

The *synovial membranes* and *synovia* are fascinating features of the joint structure. They are perfect examples of the rather 'common sense' approach to mechanics that often exists in our bodies.

The synovial membrane is a piece of soft tissue coating all of the portions of the joint ends that are covered with cartilage, especially in the gap between the bones. An exception is in the knee joint, where the synovial membrane covers only the inner area, that is, only the gap between the bones. The cartilage coats these portions of the bones and the membrane coats the cartilage. In certain joints the synovial membrane has pads containing fat that fill small gaps in the joint. The synovial membrane is quite delicate and, as a result, is subject to stress.

The synovial membrane also secretes a viscous, slippery fluid that is called *synovia* (often referred to as synovial fluid). As you can probably guess, the primary purpose of this slippery fluid is to lubricate the joint area to allow for greater smoothness of movement and less friction. Its function is not unlike that of oil on the hinges of a door.

The cells of the synovial membrane help to eliminate debris (produced by wear and tear) and any foreign substances in the area. Needless to say, the synovial membrane plays a huge role in the proper health and functioning of a synovial joint. A *bursa* is a type of synovial membrane or sac in synovial joints.

Ligaments are another protective feature of the synovial joint. These very strong, yet pliable tissues serve the important purpose of guaranteeing that there is no excessive or abnormal movement by the joint. There are ligaments that are placed inside and those that are outside of the joint socket.

Cartilaginous Joints

Cartilaginous joints are joints that are separated by larger tissue structures made of cartilage. Some of these joints eventually change into part of our skeletal structure as we get older. The majority, however, remain the same throughout life. The primary joints of this type are found in the vertebrae, the skeletal column of the spine.

The protective cartilage of many cartilaginous joints is found in the form of a disc. Ligaments are necessary for the stability of these joints. Varying degrees of movement may be allowable in this type of joint.

Fibrous Joints

Fibrous joints are those that are essentially immobile

and are connected together by fibrous tissue. Many of these joints are found in the cranium, the skeletal structure of the head area.

ARTHRITIS AND THE JOINTS

From the standpoint of arthritis, the synovial and cartilaginous joints are the ones to be most concerned with because they are the most susceptible to arthritis damage. The fact that these types of joints are able to be mobile has a great deal to do with this; not only because movement can damage the joint more easily than non-movement, but also because the problems of arthritis are most evident when a mobile joint is afflicted with damage.

The mobile joints in the body are designed, as mentioned earlier, in a very sensible manner. Each joint has a particular function that it is capable of performing provided the integrity of the joint remains structurally *and* chemically sound. Many of the joints in the body carry out what would appear to be fairly straightforward tasks such as simple arm movements, grasping, and turning the head. There are other joints that are classed as *weight-bearing joints* that carry out the rather arduous tasks of not only allowing for movement but also supporting the body's weight. Supporting body weight while movements are being carried out is particularly stressful to these joints.

Regardless of whether it is weight-bearing or not, a mobile joint will undergo a great deal of stress. The non-weight-bearing joints, although they may not have the added stress of supporting weight, often perform tasks of far greater frequency and repetition. This is particularly true of the joints in your hands. The other important factor regarding these joints is their size and structure relative to those of the weight-bearing joints. Understandably, the weight-bearing joints, such as those in your hips or knees, are much larger and have more supportive and strengthening surrounding tissue than the joints in your fingers, for instance.

The cartilaginous joints of the vertebrae are also classed as weight-bearing joints. They, as well as the hip joints, also have to compensate for your posture. No doubt you have been told, as a child or young adult, to sit up straight and not to slouch. Perhaps you were told this because it didn't 'look good' to slouch. Many of you, however, may have been warned that you would grow that way! What might have seemed a ridiculous thought even to your parents at the time has at least a shred of truth in it.

Joints are an essential part of our everyday functioning. Without them we could not carry out many of the voluntary physical tasks we take for granted every moment of our lives. Without them we could not walk, chew, bend, write, sit or perform any other structural body movement! As a result, every effort to maintain the proper functioning of the joints pays off. The parts of a body are not unlike the parts of a car: they must be taken care of and maintained in order to keep them working, otherwise they become susceptible to damage.

So how can you avoid or prevent damage to the joints in the first place? What happens when a joint or joints is already not working properly? What can you do when you have a particular disease that directly (and negatively) affects the joints? In order better to understand these issues it is important to discuss what usually goes wrong in the joint when arthritis of any type takes place.

The Mechanics of Joint Inflammation

Inflammation can occur in many other tissues in the body besides the joints. As a matter of fact, skin conditions (such as eczema) and the respiratory disorder asthma are just two well-known examples of inflammatory conditions. As mentioned, the basic definition of arthritis is 'inflammation of the joint'. The actual inflammatory process (in all forms of arthritis) has similar underlying chemical and mechanical causes; there can, however, be vast differences in what occurs prior to the inflammatory process. There are also some differences in how it will be manifested, depending to a great extent on the type of arthritis involved as well as the joint or joints affected.

So what exactly is inflammation, and how and why does it occur in the joints in the first place?

Inflammation can occur in a tissue of the body when it has become injured or damaged in some way, or if it becomes infected by a foreign substance. Inflammation of the joints is generally characterized by local swelling, tenderness, pain and perhaps a discernible warmth and redness. Of course, this is a pattern of symptoms that is familiar to us when we think of arthritis, especially the swelling and pain.

As with all the processes in the body, inflammation does not just occur out of thin air; there is a chemical process that initiates the process of inflammation and creates the symptoms. There are certain physiological occurrences that account for the symptoms:

- Local swelling is produced when the tiny capillaries in the area become more permeable – in other words, when they allow certain things to pass through them more readily than would ordinarily be the case. With inflammation, the substances that are allowed to pass through more easily are certain agents from the body's immune system.

- Redness and increased warmth in the area affected can be produced by the substantially increased blood flow to the area. The blood must flow more readily to the area in order to distribute various substances, including those directly responsible for repairing the damaged area. The increased blood flow that occurs in such cases is known as *vasodilation*, or dilation of the blood vessels.

- Precisely what produces the greatest amount of pain depends to an extent on the nature of the damage to the affected joint. The pain may at times be linked mostly to the swelling and heat. A certain inflammatory chemical called *histamine* plays a role in the local pain during inflammation, due in part to its direct effect on the nerves, and in part to the fact that it causes the swelling and heat in the first place. Eventually pain can be produced by the effect on local nerves of any actual joint deformity that may occur. In general, a combination of these factors accounts for the great physical discomfort as arthritis develops.

By far, the most interesting part of this process (if we are to understand it fully) relates to the effect of certain cells which are responsible for the inflammatory process. These cells are not only responsible for many of the symptoms associated with arthritis; they are also one of the main keys to its treatment.

These cells are related to the natural defence system of our bodies, the immune system. Our immune system is, among other things, responsible for protecting the body from harmful bacteria, viruses, cancer cells and anything that is in a place it does not belong.

The primary components of the immune system are the white blood cells. There are many classes of white blood cells and each class has its own functions.

THE MAST CELLS

One of the many types of white blood cells are called *mast cells*. They are directly responsible for the main chemical processes involved in inflammation. The mast cells are situated along blood vessels in the tissues of our body. While other white blood cells spend their time patrolling the bloodstream, the mast cells find their location particularly conducive to their primary function. By maintaining a position along the vascular system of bodily tissues, they are much closer to where they have to work.

So how does a little mast cell cause all of this agonizing inflammation?

A mast cell chemically induces inflammation due to the fact that:

a It causes the release of *histamine* locally in the tissues

b It causes the release of *leukotrienes*, (another inflammatory chemical)

c It is also responsible for the activity of inflammatory *prostaglandins*

d It produces other chemical mediators of inflammation including those that cause *chemotaxis* (chemotaxis is a process in which mast cell-derived chemicals attract 'attacking' white blood cells into the affected area)

HISTAMINE

Histamine is a chemical whose name is probably already familiar to you. When you have an allergic reaction such as hayfever, what do you take? An anti-histamine. The reason why an anti-histamine works to suppress the symptoms of an allergy such as hayfever is that histamine produces the symptoms. This type of reaction is also inflammatory in nature.

Histamine and its related chemical, *bradykinin*, account directly for local swelling, pain, redness and warmth in the affected areas of arthritis. As mentioned, histamine is released by the mast cells. It is not completely clear what activates the inflammation, but various substances released due to damage in the joints appear to be the main instigators. This process is speeded up if any of the released substances activate a white blood cell 'red alert'.

Remember, the white blood cells, such as the mast cells, are components of the immune system. The immune system is most active in areas infiltrated by foreign substances. When damage occurs to joint tissue, certain substances that will be considered 'invaders' by the immune cells may be released. Such substances are known as *antigens*. Certain types of immune cells then take on the task of destroying them.

LEUKOTRIENES

Leukotrienes can be over a thousand times more inflammatory than even histamine. The leukotrienes that mast cells release are particularly important in the healing process and account for a great deal of the pain experienced in the affected area. One specific leukotriene called LTB4 appears to be especially notorious for its undesirable effects. Leukotrienes are created as a result of *fatty acids* derived from fats in the diet. The specific type of fatty acid responsible for the severely inflammatory leukotrienes is called *arachidonic acid*. Arachidonic acid is a polyunsaturated fatty acid found primarily in animal fats (although it can be manufactured in the body from certain non-animal fats). Leukotrienes are created when this fatty acid is exposed to oxygen in the body. The effect of a person's diet on leukotrienes will be covered more comprehensively at several points throughout the later chapters of this book. As is the case with histamine, leukotrienes are natural and necessary chemicals of the body.

Any chemical used up by the body must then be replaced, and all chemicals in the body are dependent on whatever is needed to make them. Histamines, leukotrienes and prostaglandins are no exceptions to this rule. In Chapters Two and Four we will discuss which factors cause an increase in these chemicals, as well as measures that can be utilized to decrease their production. Needless to say, manipulating the supply of such agents would have a considerable effect on inflammation.

PROSTAGLANDINS

In order to activate certain inflammatory responses and augment the effects of chemicals such as bradykinin and histamine, another class of inflammatory substances is needed. *Prostaglandins* are actually hormone-like chemicals that, like leukotrienes, are produced from fats. Prostaglandins regulate inflammatory activity. Certain prostaglandins produce a substantially increased inflammatory response; others have the opposite effect. The most inflammatory type is *prostaglandin E2 (PGE2)*.

Prostaglandin E2, like the inflammatory leukotrienes, is produced from arachidonic acid metabolism. Arachidonic acid has certain storage sites that the body uses as an 'emergency supply'. When an emergency occurs, such as joint damage or even an infection, arachidonic acid is released from storage and is converted into PGE2. In the case of an infection, the newly produced PGE2 increases the body temperature (e.g. fever) in order to rid the body of the infection. In the case of joint damage, PGE2 causes inflammation. Interestingly, as you will find later, prostaglandins are among the most important aspects of arthritis *treatment* as well as its development.

Inflammation: The Benefits

So why does mast cell-induced inflammation have to happen? This is a valid question, especially when you consider the fact that the mast cells do not actually attack invaders themselves. Among the main reasons why the mast cells carry out their inflammatory action in the joints are:

- Vasodilation (redness and warmth) and the increased capillary permeability (local swelling) allow for easier distribution of 'invader-destroying' white blood cells.
- Certain chemicals released serve to signal or attract the invader-destroying white blood cells to the affected area.

The pain and tenderness actually serve to discourage the person from moving or using the affected joint. This theoretically prevents further damage and allows for quicker healing or repair to take place. Also, the pain alerts us to the fact that there is something very wrong in the affected area. You must admit, there is no better way to make a person take notice! Local swelling helps to cushion and partially immobilize the affected joint, in order to restrict use. These effects promote a better environment for protection and repair.

As you can see, while chemicals such as histamine and leukotrienes represent most of what we consider so intolerable about arthritis, the process is (in its own irritating way) necessary. This is one of the most difficult aspects of the body's protective functioning to accept. It must be remembered that if any of these necessary processes were missing, we would not be able to carry out even the simplest healing process. Nor would we know, at least until it might be too late, that there was anything wrong.

All of the naturally occurring chemicals in the body play some essential role, no matter how non-essential their effect may seem. Inflammation is certainly no exception. As a result, any 'raw materials' required to manufacture these chemicals must be deemed essential as well. You may already be aware of many of these essential raw materials that make the more obviously important body chemicals: for instance, essential vitamins and minerals. We also need certain fatty acids to function, and arachidonic acid is one of them – no matter how dastardly it appears on the surface! Therefore, according to its scientific and medical definition, arachidonic acid is an *essential fatty acid (EFA)*.

Inflammation: The Negative Side

You are probably already reciting to yourself a long list of what you *personally* know to be the negative side of inflammation. Nevertheless, there are other concerns besides the obvious symptomatic ones that you should be aware of. While it is important and perhaps even somewhat comforting to know that the *intended* function of inflammation is basically good and necessary, it is also vital to understand that there is a substantial 'diminishing return' to this process over time.

Basically, inflammation is a protective process that has presumably always existed in animal species such as humans. The scientifically-determined, intended purpose of inflammation, at least where the joints are concerned, relates to protecting joint tissues against acute injury or naturally occurring day-to-day damage.

When the inflammatory process is activated by either an acute 'one-off' injury or day-to-day strain, it is generally perfectly capable of averting any permanent problem. It is usually only when there is prolonged or repeated damage that things begin to go wrong. The situation is a bit like that in an emergency unit at a hospital. As long as the patients are brought in in small numbers and there is plenty of time between patients, the doctors and staff will have no major difficulties dealing with them. If the patients take longer than expected to treat, however, or if they are coming in too frequently, then there will be problems taking care of them all. Consider also what would happen if each injury sustained by the people waiting to be treated were getting worse and worse as time passed by!

This brings us to one further aspect of inflammation that has not yet been discussed: a little known chemical reaction that occurs as a result of inflammation. Over a short time this reaction doesn't amount to much, but over the long term it has severe implications. This process involves agents called *lysosomal enzymes*.

In order to understand these enzymes we need to go back to the information about the synovial membrane.

As you will recall, the synovial membrane cushions and protects the ends of the joints in the space between the bones, where they would otherwise meet. This protection is carried out not only by the actual tissue of the membrane but also by any enclosed fat pads and the joint-lubricating synovial fluid. The synovial membrane also carries out another natural process that occurs in response to tissue damage. It releases lysosomal enzymes from its cells. Lysosomal enzymes break down debris and foreign matter, which are plentiful at the site of injury. This is a very positive activity, but unfortunately these enzymes also carry out a destructive purpose as well. The enzymes are potent and can digest many different substances. Unfortunately they inadvertently begin to break down the cartilage and bone structure in the area where released. As you can probably guess, this does untold additional damage to the joint.

It is clear that the longer the inflammatory process lasts, the more lysosomal enzymes are actively going to destroy not only the soft but also the hard tissue of the joint. This is also a problem when there is short-term but repetitive injury to the same area. A good example of this is sports injuries. Other than the symptoms themselves, lysosomal enzymes represent the major concern in the inflammatory process of joint damage.

Knowing all this about inflammatory process leads many to the understandable conclusion that the main priority in arthritis should be to try to avoid inflammation. However, considering what you now know about the purpose of inflammation, it should be clear that this is perhaps not conducive to the short-term healing benefits of the process. What a dilemma! As you know, whenever you have a dilemma the best way to solve it is usually some sort of compromise. The logical compromise here would be for the inflammatory response to be as short as possible in order to allow for the short-term healing *without* the long-term lysosomal enzyme damage. The problem is, *you* may be willing to compromise but the arthritis is not. Arthritis is a *chronic* or semi-chronic condition in essentially all cases; if you leave it up to the natural course of events, the arthritis will be self-perpetuating. This may sound quite ominous, but do not be too disappointed. There are effective and scientifically researched methods of addressing this problem. (These will be discussed in later chapters.)

Although there are issues such as those mentioned above that are relevant to all forms of arthritis to one extent or another, it is important to have an understanding of the specific type of arthritis you may be suffering with. This way the cause can be better identified in a particular case and treatment can include the cause as well as the symptoms. The next chapter outlines the most common forms of arthritis, to help you to get a picture of what is likely to be going on in your joints. It will also allow you to better understand the preventive and treatment approaches that will be discussed in Chapters Three and Four.

PLEASE NOTE: Although the following chapter will provide you with information that will help in the diagnosis of the different arthritic conditions, if you have not been diagnosed already, it is recommended that you discuss the matter with a qualified medical health practitioner. In order for diagnosis of certain arthritic disorders (such as rheumatoid arthritis) to be accurate to the highest possible degree, certain tests may need to be performed.

CHAPTER 2

The Various Forms of Arthritis

It must be stressed again just how important it is to identify properly what type of arthritis you have. This will help not only with assessing the likely development of your condition, it will also make any treatment measures more specific and, consequently, more effective. Without the benefit of proper identification we are left with only the universal symptoms to treat. This may not seem so bad, as many arthritis sufferers are perhaps only concerned with the immediate symptoms; however, it is always better to know as much as possible about what ails you.

Ironically, general knowledge about arthritis can make a person concentrate less on learning about the individual type he or she has. Perhaps a great deal of this can be blamed on the heavy marketing of over-the-counter medication for the treatment of arthritis symptoms. When people are encouraged simply to buy a bottle of aspirin, for instance, they are unlikely to dig any deeper into their particular problem. Sufferers of various health disorders are naturally attracted to a 'magic bullet' which, if only temporarily, suppresses their pain. But these magic bullets do nothing to help the *cause* of their suffering. Side-effects are common as well. This does not mean that symptoms should not be addressed. It just means that much more emphasis should be put on:

a Treating the cause
b Utilizing research-proven treatments of symptoms with fewer side-effects or risks (including many natural methods)
c Using preventive approaches. (As mentioned, the only *guaranteed* cure of any disease or disorder is *prevention*!)

OSTEOARTHRITIS

Osteoarthritis may not be the most well-known form of arthritis, but it is by far the most common: it has been estimated that more than 75 per cent of adults over the age of 50 have it!

Osteoarthritis is also known as *degenerative joint disease*. This should give you some clue as to the serious nature of this condition and its progression. Although 'wear and tear' over-simplifies what actually occurs, it is a fairly accurate description of its development and a typical cause, and helps to explain why it is so common in adults over 50. Wear and tear does not, however, account for all the causes involved. The popular misconception is that wear and tear is the only factor, which is why few people consider it realistic to try and prevent its occurrence and those who already have it tend to resign themselves to its continued development.

As long as this misconception endures we will see the disastrous effects of osteoarthritis in a high percentage of people. It is important to understand two points:

1 Normal degeneration of a joint is *not* the only factor involved (as a matter of fact, in optimal health the body is designed to repair the effects of such wear reasonably well)

2 Much of the wear and tear is either speeded up or
   even in some cases *caused* by other controllable
   factors which hinder repair mechanisms

The symptoms of osteoarthritis are similar from
person to person, yet they vary somewhat depending
on which joints are affected and how long the condition
has progressed. A list of the more common symptoms
includes:

- Joint pain and tenderness
- Joint stiffness, especially after rest
- Chronic cracking or grinding of joints
- Local swelling
- Pain brought on by overuse
- Progressive immobility due to joint degeneration and
  deformity

This condition can affect many different joints in the
body, but the ones usually affected are the hips, knees,
spinal joints and the hands.

Now let us look in more depth at the development of
osteoarthritis and its common symptoms.

The Development of Osteoarthritis

As one might expect, the main priority of the sufferer in
osteoarthritis is probably the symptoms. This is not
exclusive to arthritis; it probably pertains to most health
disorders. Most people consider the symptoms in terms
of treatment, but it must be remembered that they are
also important to diagnosis. Because there are so many
conditions put under the general heading of arthritis,
this makes the symptoms an even more important tool
in proper identification. The chronic symptoms listed

above are very common in osteoarthritis sufferers.

Any joint pain experienced has more than one cause. The reasons behind various common inflammatory problems were listed in Chapter One. It was mentioned that general inflammatory mechanisms included a sort of local 'pain-activating factor'. This mechanism is dependent on inflammatory chemicals such as histamine. When histamine (or the related chemical bradykinin) is released locally in osteoarthritic tissues, certain 'pain fibres' become activated, thereby producing joint pain. Presumably this mechanism is intended to discourage movement and to act as a signal that there is something wrong. Even if there were no such activation of the pain fibres, the pressure and heat experienced in an affected joint would likely produce some discomfort anyway.

In osteoarthritis there is a particularly disturbing cause of the local pain. This cause is not exclusive to osteoarthritis but it is perhaps more severe than in many other forms of arthritis. The cause is actual damage to the joint. In osteoarthritis it is often the case that the joint damage itself causes many of the arthritis symptoms (such as inflammation), rather than their first being caused by some other factor(s). In many other types of arthritis the symptoms (such as inflammation, pain, etc.) often present before there is significant wear and tear from use.

So what is the significance of this difference? Either way there is a problem, but a particularly unfortunate implication of osteoarthritis is clear. When symptoms do not occur until the joint tissue has already been significantly damaged, then healing is a great deal more difficult. Certain other types of arthritis have even more insidious and disturbing characteristics, but at least you often have the 'early warning' symptoms before large-scale tissue destruction has taken place.

Besides the above considerations, the joints most frequently affected by osteoarthritis are required constantly for even the most conservative of day-to-day functioning; as a result, avoiding further wear and tear is just not practical.

In osteoarthritis, this damage is experienced in hard tissue (e.g. bone) as well as soft. This causes an alteration in the bone structure in the joint. Even in the early stages, before the hard tissue is as significantly affected, the wearing away of the synovial tissue (if applicable) or the cartilage starts to eliminate the smooth and unimpeded mechanical integrity of the joint. Once the soft, protective tissue is worn away in an area, two seemingly opposite effects can occur. First, the space between the bone ends closes and the bone ends start grinding against one another. Conversely, if local swelling is extreme this can push the joint ends even further apart, thereby altering the 'perfect fit' of the joint.

As it turns out, local swelling is not generally as prominent in osteoarthritis as it is in certain other types of arthritis, so the first scenario is especially common. As you can probably imagine, when the bones have been grinding together for a while there is little mobility left. When movement *does* occur, the pain can be excruciating! This is especially true upon waking or after excessive use.

In spite of all this, the human body is incredibly resilient. It seems to have a protective measure for almost any problem. For instance, if you break your leg or fracture any bone in your body, your body begins the healing process by repairing the bone by manufacturing new bone material at the point of fracture. The protective measure against the wearing away of bone tissue at joint ends is much the same, but while the process works very well for repairing a fracture, primarily because most fractures do not change the shape, size and continuity of bone, this is unfortunately not true of osteoarthritis damage. The loss of bone is not manifested as a 'clean break'. In addition, the damage may be done faster than the healing process can compensate for. As a result of all this, what often constitutes joint-end repair turns out to be very unhelpful lumps, bumps or spurs of calcified hard tissue called *osteophytes*. These osteophytes, which are often known as bone spurs, certainly do *not* represent a perfect replica of the original joint, and as a result they often account for even more pain and immobility. In severe cases, where the joint ends are making constant contact along the joint margins, the bone ends may virtually fuse together – which would, of course, put an end to mobility.

Although the development of osteoarthritis can vary somewhat from person to person, it typically follows the progression outlined above. This news is very depressing and disconcerting at face value. It also becomes clear to those who learn of its true characteristics that, under ordinary circumstances, the chances of reversing any of the damage or even halting the development of osteoporosis seems highly unrealistic. It must be said that the primary intention of this book is *not* to perpetuate a feeling of helplessness in osteoarthritis sufferers. Actually, quite the opposite is true! There is a great deal of medical and scientific research which proves that there are safe, natural and effective methods which can be used either to prevent, relieve the symptoms of, halt the progression of, or, in some cases, even reverse some or a great deal of the damage caused by osteoarthritis. Those suffering the earlier stages of its development can expect the greatest chance of reversal and prevention of new damage. It is true that there are some cases where the joint deformity and immobility are beyond any significant correction, but even in these cases prevention of any worsening as well as reduction of symptoms (without side-effects) may well be achieved. Whether less severe or more severe, obtaining the proper information is the first step to either significant or, at worst, partial control over the problem. The information to help prevent, treat the symptoms of, and/or reverse damage caused by osteoarthritis will follow in later chapters. Now let us look at the parts of the body typically affected by this condition.

Body Parts Affected

As mentioned, the following are the most common joints or areas affected by osteoarthritis:

• hips
• knees
• spine
• hands

When we look at the parts of the body that are generally affected most by osteoarthritis, a telling pattern emerges. The hips, knees and spine are classified as 'weight-bearing joints'. Weight-bearing joints are so named because they assume the brunt of the responsibility for supporting a person's weight, especially during movement. The weight of the body is more easily supported by a person's skeleton and muscles when there is no movement and when the supporting joints are not bent. When movement such as walking takes place, the stress of the weight becomes distributed more exclusively on the supporting joints.

THE HIP

The hip is a perfect example of a highly stressed joint. It is a 'ball and socket' type of joint. As a result of this structure, the hip joint is an exact fit; any alteration in its shape would present significant problems. The hips not only support the weight of the upper half of your body, they are also subjected to considerable motion-induced stress. As mentioned in Chapter One, each joint has its own intended range of movement. The hips are one of the joints with the greatest range and, as such, must compensate for this.

Hips are also subjected to some of the most frequent and jarring movements. The combination of supporting much of your weight and bearing wide-ranging, frequent and intense movement causes the hips to be a major target of wear and tear. Even if the body does not happen to be moving at the time, there is still the issue of posture. As the body was intended to use a strong base to help support its weight, if the upper body is slouched, bent or curved this puts more pressure on the hip joints and the surrounding muscle.

The hips may be susceptible to significant pounding, but the design of the body tends to compensate for much of this stress. In the case of the hips, part of the compensation is covered in the mere size of the joint involved. Fortunately the hip joint is large and, as such, the protective tissue is relatively strong and proportionately large in size. The cartilage, ligaments and synovial membrane are fairly substantial and the joint is surrounded by plenty of supporting muscle tissue (*see*

Figure 1.1.).

In spite of all this size, padding and support, eventually the hip joint can buckle under the pressure. Because of the huge responsibility of the hips, any damage to this joint has severe consequences. Every effort must be made to preserve its integrity and function.

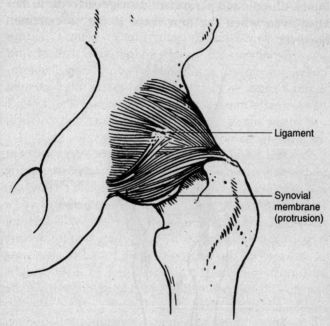

Figure 1.1. THE HIP JOINT

THE KNEE

The knee is another common joint to be damaged by osteoarthritis. The knee is classified as a hinge-type synovial joint. It most certainly is a weight-bearing joint, but unlike the hips it does not have nearly so much help and support to carry out its tasks. Fortunately the knees do not have quite the range of movement that the hip joints have. The knee is obviously restricted: it can move no further forward once straight (hyper-extension), but it still is allowed to make slight movements laterally. Any forceable effort to hyper-extend the knee or move the joint too far laterally are probably the most common causes of acute knee injury. Chronic and permanent damage can occur to the knee even when the movement is not so extreme, however.

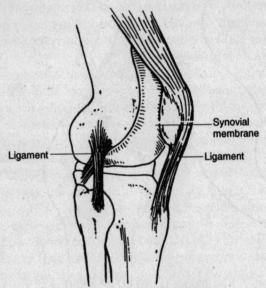

Figure 1.2. THE KNEE JOINT

When you look at the structure of a knee joint (*See Figure 1.2.*), it seems inconceivable that fairly normal movement could damage it. The knee has the most extensive network of synovial tissue in the body. However, even if there is not much improper movement, if the protective tissue is damaged by other means, osteoarthritis can still set in.

THE SPINE

Clearly the joints of the vertebrae are among the most vital in the body for many reasons. They are not only part of the column that supports the upper body and provides a place for the ribs to go. The vertebrae also protect the spinal cord – the vital link between the brain and the body. The vertebral column is a mixture of cartilaginous and synovial joints. One of the best-known features of these joints are the discs which separate and cushion them (*See Figure 1.3.*).

Healthy spinal discs are the key to a healthy and properly functioning vertebral column. Unfortunately, they are not immune to destruction. As with knee joints, it does not always take improper movement or bad posture to damage the protective tissue of the vertebral joints. Other factors that can harm them will be discussed shortly. Suffice it to say, the spinal joints are a primary target for osteoarthritis, due in part to the unending mechanical stress they endure.

The vertebral discs are made of cartilage tissue and they provide essential protection to the vertebral joints. They are somewhat similar to the brake pads in a car. If they wear away you have things grinding together which should not. At a certain point this grinding produces irreparable damage. As with brakes, if there is no pad, it is just a matter of time before the two sides fuse together and lock. Of course, you can always have your brakes replaced. Where your spinal joint ends are concerned, this is not a viable proposition.

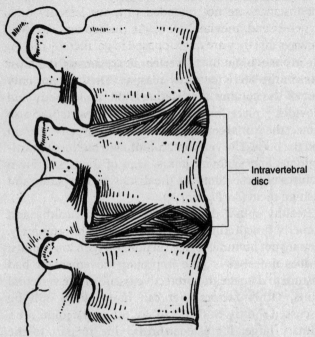

Figure 1.3. THE VERTEBRAL JOINTS

THE HANDS

The hands are a slightly different story where osteoarthritis is concerned. First of all, they obviously do not
contain weight-bearing joints. Secondly, unlike the hips,
knees and spine, they are not directly affected by the
posture or integrity of other joints in the body. In what
way, then, are the joints of the hands similar to the weight-
bearing joints in terms of the risk of osteoarthritis?

The hands contain some of the most highly used
joints in the body (*see Figure 1.4.*). Because we gain so
much dexterity in their use, we tend to utilize them
almost unconsciously. As a result they are frequently

overworked and abused. The middle joints in the fingers, for instance, are not intended to move laterally or to hyper-extend. Inevitably they are pushed and stretched in ways that they are not supposed to go, thereby putting stress on their stabilizing tissues. Excessive and improper use of any mobile joint can allow osteoarthritis to set in, even if it is not a weight-bearing joint.

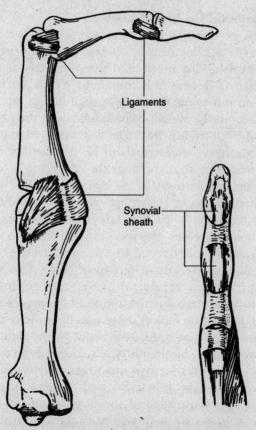

Figure 1.4. THE JOINTS OF THE FINGERS

The finger joints are supported by ligaments, flexor tendons and synovial membrane tissue. The fingers have built-in protective measures to restrict movement to the intended range, but chronic stress can weaken all the supporting tissues. This accounts to a great extent for the fact that the fingers are a common visible target of other types of arthritis as well.

Osteoarthritis: The Likely Causes

There is no question that wear and tear plays a major role in the development of osteoarthritis. This certainly helps explain why more than three-quarters of adults over 50 will develop this condition. We all put untold stress on our joints throughout each day of our lives, especially on the weight-bearing joints and the joints of the hands. Obviously the longer we have lived, the more stress we have subjected them to. It is getting to the point where we should change the old saying to 'death, taxes, *and* osteoarthritis' as the sure things in this world.

Perhaps the most bizarre fact about this condition is that it has become the rule rather than the exception. How many diseases can you think of that are not at least relatively abnormal in their occurrence? Even heart disease does not affect most of us. This makes osteoarthritis a very strange disorder to analyse. Usually, when trying to determine all the possible causes of a disease you look at those who have the condition and find out what is different about them; their background, lifestyle, biochemistry, etc. This is more difficult with osteoarthritis for two main reasons: normal wear and tear is not the only factor, and you end up analysing a huge percentage of the population, made up primarily of people with similar backgrounds, average biochemistry and presumably average health, trying to find something abnormal about them! How can you take a *normal* group of people comprising much of the population and find something *abnormal* about them? In spite of this dilemma, certain trends *have* been noted in osteoarthritis sufferers.

WEAR AND TEAR

Undoubtedly this is beginning to sound like a broken record, as this term has popped up again and again. There is good reason for this. Like it or not, wear and tear is indeed a major factor in osteoarthritis, although it is by no means the *only* factor. If you have been using the same knees or the same hips for 60 years, there is bound to be some damage! To use a rather predictable analogy, you cannot drive your car for ever without replacing the tyres occasionally.

Since there is no practical way to avoid the normal wear of the joints through ordinary stresses of movement and body weight support, all you can hope to do is try to lessen the load and repair the damage more efficiently. As far as wear and tear is concerned, supporting *excessive* weight will only make matters worse. The added stress of overweight or obesity is damaging to all the weight-bearing joints. The protective tissue of such joints will most likely be worn out much more quickly, partly due to the greater compression of the joint space.

In osteoarthritis, the progressive reduction in the joint space is primarily the result of the loss of the protective tissue residing in the space. This damage occurs throughout life as a result of use but, *under optimal circumstances*, your body has mechanisms designed to repair such damage and more or less restore normal

joint integrity. Such optimal circumstances will be
discussed in later chapters.

Osteoarthritic damage is not always age-driven.
Another aspect of wear and tear can come about quite
accidentally. We now know that normal wear and tear
is only likely to present an osteoarthritic problem after
many decades of use. But what about when wear and
tear is accelerated by abnormal use? A perfect example
of this is chronic injury. With a 'one-off' injury, the
repair processes of the body are fairly efficient at re-
creating a normal joint. For instance, if you injure your
ankle while walking or hurt your knee while exercising,
as long as you rest the injured area it usually heals up
nicely in time. However, if you happen to re-injure the
same ankle or knee several times, the chances of it
being *properly* repaired may diminish each time. Sometimes even with one-off injuries there can be improper
healing. This is especially likely if there was not ample
rest and healing time. In either case, osteoarthritic
damage can set in even if you are comparatively young.
This is not as likely to manifest badly soon after it happens, but as time goes on, normal wear, and a reduced
ability to repair cartilage take their toll. As a result, the
once chronically injured joint is likely to be trouble.

Ageing and Collagen Matrix Repair
There are many factors relevant to joint repair. One of them
pertains to age. It is easy to understand the correlation
between age and joint damage, at least from the standpoint
of wear and tear. However, the fact that you may have been
putting weight on the same knees for a longer period of time
is not the only relevant detail to growing older.

As we grow older there seems to be a diminished ability to repair connective tissue in general in the body.

The connective tissue areas that are very susceptible to this diminished state of health include, among others, the vascular (blood vessel) system, the skin, the bones and, of course, the joints. Very seldom do any of us take the time to think of how many blood vessels we must have in our body, or perhaps how much of our body is made of skin. Yet these are only two of the many categories of tissue that are in constant need of repair. By repair, we mean what is known as a *collagen matrix*.

Collagen is a type of protein which acts to help bond connective tissue cells together. Collagen is a primary constituent of joint-protecting tissues. It is also the main component of the non-mineral matrix of the bones, the skin, and the blood vessels (veins, arteries, capillaries). If the available collagen (and other parts of the matrix) is having to be used to repair all of these tissues and many more, then the ability to repair *significant* damage to any of them is obviously greatly impaired. If we look at the high incidence of cardiovascular disease and osteoporosis (brittle, porous bones) as well as of osteoarthritis in countries that follow a 'Western' lifestyle and diet, it is clear that there is often more than one area significantly damaged in the same person. From the standpoint of an osteoarthritis sufferer, this is a substantial setback to the speed of joint repair. After all, whatever repair materials are going to the blood vessels, bones or the skin are *not* going to the joints. What makes matters worse in the case of osteoarthritis is the fact that even more repair of cartilage and other protective tissue is needed because the joints being damaged are often so large to begin with.

The good news is that there is something that can be done to speed up the repair process *and* to slow down the progression of the damage. In order to understand

how such benefits might be gained, you need to understand the mechanisms (other than wear and tear) causing the damage.

Free Radicals, Lysosomal Enzymes and Bacterial Activity

FREE RADICALS

The subject of free radicals is quite an extensive one,
but there are certain points particularly relevant to
osteoarthritis. Free radicals are molecules which travel
through the body and can damage or interfere with
proper cellular function and development. Free radicals
come in many different types, and can come from many
different sources, both external and internal. Many of
them are produced by the body during its normal metabolic processes. The external sources of free radicals that
most people are familiar with are those that come from
air pollution, cigarette smoke, car exhaust, sun exposure and the like. It seems that two of the free radical
types that are particularly notorious for their damaging
effects in arthritis are *superoxides* and *peroxides*.

Free radicals of the superoxide variety are not really
avoidable. Among other sources they are often
produced in the body in a natural process whereby
certain ordinary body chemicals are *oxidized* ('oxidized'
refers to the process whereby substances are exposed
and degraded by oxygen). Also, superoxide radicals are
used by certain white blood cells as a sort of poison to
kill invading bacteria. In spite of their often 'natural'
origin, superoxide radicals interfere with the proper
development of collagen matrix and cause existing
protective tissue to be damaged prematurely. In addition, superoxides appear to be a contributing factor in
the destruction of synovial lubricating fluid.

The peroxide free radicals are produced in a process whereby unsaturated fats are affected by oxygen. Rancid oil is an example of this 'denaturing' of unsaturated fats by oxygen. This process is greatly accelerated by heat. As a result, cooked oils and especially fried foods are substantial sources of peroxide radicals. Peroxides are not just formed in a bottle or in a frying pan, however, they are also produced in the body when fats are metabolized.

Whether consumed in the diet or manufactured in the body (and perhaps even locally in the joint area), peroxides, like superoxides, can damage and inhibit repair of joint tissue and lubricating fluid. At least some of the destruction of certain joints is caused by the fact that free radical damage can stimulate the release of lysosomal enzymes from local cells.

Oxygen is one of the great dichotomies of life. On the one hand, it is absolutely necessary for us to live. On the other hand, it leads to the destruction of the life-giving cells of our body. It does this by producing various forms of free radicals such as superoxides and peroxides. This destructive effect does not just pertain to the cells of the joints, it can pertain to any cells. In Chapter Four we will discuss how to reduce free radical-induced damage to the joints.

LYSOSOMAL ENZYMES

The importance of lysosomal enzymes in osteoarthritis development cannot be overstated. You may recall that these enzymes are actually released by the cells of the synovial membrane itself in many joints of the body. This release is generally a reaction to inflammation. The lysosomal enzymes are capable of digesting a huge range of substances in an attempt to rid the area of debris. Unfortunately, included on this list of substances are cartilage and bone tissue. If active for long periods in a joint, the lysosomal enzymes advance any damage that has already taken place. The inflammation, which is supposed to be so protective in the short term, becomes quite destructive in the long term.

BACTERIAL ACTIVITY

It has frequently been suggested that various micro-organisms may play a damaging part in the development of arthritis. Considering what we already know about the role of the immune system in inflammatory response, the possible negative effect of bacteria is not at all far-fetched.

When invading bacteria are identified and attacked by immune cells, certain processes can take place. In one scenario, antibodies (made by the white blood cells from the bone marrow) may become attached to the bacteria; other white blood cells will then move in to attack and destroy these invaders. In another scenario, the bacteria may be destroyed by white blood cells without the intervention of an antibody.

If either scenario takes place in the joints on a large scale, inflammation is bound to occur. This, in turn, starts a magnified process that may involve lysosomal enzymes, superoxides and hydrogen peroxide radicals, with the end result an accelerated destruction of joint tissue and/or impairment to the creation of new cartilage.

Older Women, Younger Men and Osteoarthritis

The most blatant risk factor in osteoarthritis development is something that we have absolutely *no* control over: our age and gender. It appears that in the 'over

50' age group, women have approximately a *ten-fold* risk of osteoarthritis! Even more strange is the fact that when the condition occurs in those younger than their mid-forties, they are much more likely to be men. It is difficult to know exactly why these seemingly opposite statistics exist, but there is at least one factor that definitely springs to mind when considering the risk in older women: osteoporosis.

You may be familiar with the term *osteoporosis*. It is a condition that results when the bones become extremely porous and brittle. Most cases of osteoporosis occur in women past the age of 50 who are going through or who are past the menopause. Certain factors make older women more susceptible to osteoporosis. The more common cause is the reduction in oestrogen that leads to an increase in the breakdown of bone by parathyroid hormone and the reduced utilization of the mineral calcium.

Calcium is the mineral that is most needed in building bones. It is not the *only* element needed in bone building, however. The *collagen matrix* of the bone is important as well. The fact that collagen matrix is significantly damaged in both osteoarthritis and osteoporosis may give us a clue as to one of the correlations between older women and a high risk of osteoarthritis. As mentioned, if the need for available collagen matrix materials in the joints is being 'shared' with another degenerative condition, then there will be problems. After all, we do not have an unending supply of collagen matrix materials, and the joints are likely to pay a big price for any deficiency. That price could be osteoarthritis.

This is not to say that all women over 50 are riddled with osteoporosis and thus will have osteoarthritis.

However, one thing should be reiterated: research seems to show that women going through the oestrogen reduction that occurs automatically with menopause have a reduced bone density due to increased breakdown by parathyroid hormone. This may increase the body's requirement of the necessary bone-repairing constituents, including collagen.

A correlation between osteoarthritis and osteoporosis is perhaps too significant to ignore, yet more research needs to be done to help draw definitive conclusions as to why women are so much more prone to osteoarthritis than men near or after the age of 50. Collagen matrix repair problems do *not* occur only in women, however, and it must be remembered that men younger than in their mid-forties are more likely to have osteoarthritis than women of the same age.

Dietary and Lifestyle Factors

At times it can be difficult to accept the incredible control that diet and lifestyle have over our general state of health. Nevertheless, with each new research study, it becomes more obvious that this control encompasses most every health disorder. Rather than being depressed about such data, we should be glad that this information is surfacing. After all, it often represents our main source of hope – *we can actually control our own health* – that is, *if* we heed the advice offered by the research. In Chapter Four we will discuss how nutritional and lifestyle factors play a role in the development and in the treatment and/or prevention of osteoarthritis.

To review, the body's requirement for collagen matrix repair in osteoarthritis may greatly increase when:

a Wear and tear in certain joints builds up with age
b Cartilage synthesis is reduced with age
c Cartilage and protective tissues are damaged due to free radicals, lysosomal enzymes and/or bacterial activity
d Chronic injury to joint occurs
e Collagen matrix capability is being shared with another degenerative disease affecting connective tissue
f Certain dietary and lifestyle factors reduce cartilage and protective tissue synthesis

Regardless of what factor or factors are responsible for a person's osteoarthritis, it is vital to know what can be done about it. It is also extremely important to be familiar with the possible links between diet/ lifestyle and osteoarthritis. Many of these factors may greatly increase the risk of development and even speed of destruction of osteoarthritis. On the other hand, there are many natural and very safe methods of preventing and treating both the symptoms and causes of osteoarthritis. Many of these methods have clinically proven benefits that have been published in medical and scientific journals of research. These methods include, among other things, the use of vitamins, minerals, herbs, enzymes and other natural or nutritional substances, as well as changing your diet as necessary. Many of these methods will be outlined in Chapter Four.

Remember, proper diagnosis is vital for the best results in any health or medical programme. If you have not had a diagnosis of your particular form of arthritis, it is recommended that you consult a qualified medical health practitioner.

RHEUMATOID ARTHRITIS

Rheumatoid arthritis is without question one of the most debilitating and destructive of all health disorders. Although you are probably quite familiar with its name, thankfully it is not nearly as common as osteoarthritis. As you know, osteoarthritis is likely to affect the vast majority of the population at some point, at least in countries with a 'Westernized' approach to diet and lifestyle. Rheumatoid arthritis appears to affect less than 5 per cent of the population (approximately 2 per cent may be likely). As with osteoarthritis, women are the unfortunate sufferers in most cases. As a matter of fact, women are between two and three times more likely to develop this disease.

Rheumatoid arthritis illustrates perfectly the problem of using the generic term 'arthritis'. Rheumatoid arthritis is certainly a form of arthritis, but in spite of having some recognizable arthritic symptoms, it is quite different from various other forms. These differences, as you will find out, are not at all minor.

The insidious and highly self-perpetuating nature of rheumatoid arthritis makes early identification extremely important. Because the most obvious symptom is representative of general arthritic complaints with which people are familiar, sufferers are more inclined to consider an 'official' diagnosis unnecessary. Nothing could be further from the truth! Although symptom patterns can be a useful tool in diagnosing rheumatoid arthritis, diagnosis beyond a reasonable doubt may require further and specialized testing procedures. Perhaps more than any other form, a proper diagnosis and prompt treatment are essential in rheumatoid arthritis.

The substantial research into this disease has shown that it is most likely an *auto-immune disorder*. The term 'auto-immune' refers to a situation in which a person's immune system mistakenly perceives *normal* body cells to be invaders. This has most disastrous implications for any parts of the body containing such cells. Auto-immunity will be elaborated on below.

Another of the more disturbing characteristics of rheumatoid arthritis that differs from other forms has to do with its long-term development. First of all, where osteoarthritis is much more common in those over 50 or so, rheumatoid arthritis can develop at any point in life. It typically will begin when a person is in his or her twenties or thirties. The manifestation of this condition can last a lifetime, or it can last a matter of a few months or years.

A condition such as osteoarthritis will typically affect only those joints that are weakened by wear and tear, injury or some other cause of damage or stress. With rheumatoid arthritis, *all* joints may be affected over the course of time. The joints in the body that typically manifest the condition in the earlier stages are the smaller ones. In general, the most affected joints include those in the fingers, toes, knees, elbows, wrists, ankles and shoulders, but then the condition progresses to other joints. Problems in non-joint tissue (such as the skin) may be associated with rheumatoid arthritis as well.

Inflammation in the affected joints is typically much more severe than in osteoarthritis, and the disease usually develops in a symmetrical manner. In other words, if the fingers are affected, the condition will be basically the same on both hands. This pattern should apply to any joint affected in the early stages. Although the disease spreads to different joints throughout its progression, it will often show up in several joints early on.

We tend to associate arthritis in general with only the inflammation of and/or damage to the joints. Once again rheumatoid arthritis differs in this, displaying its own unique characteristics. In the earlier stages of its development there may be very mild or vague symptoms in the joints, but also fatigue or weakness and perhaps a mild fever. As with osteoarthritis, eventually the damage to the joints can be extreme. In rheumatoid arthritis, obvious visible joint deformity is common over time.

Another disparity is the fact that the condition does not *always* spread or get worse. In fact, people occasionally enter an apparent 'spontaneous remission'. In such cases, the rheumatoid arthritis appears to cease to do damage or produce further symptoms, sometimes indefinitely. What often happens, however, is that if remission occurs it will only be temporary; the condition will continue to go through phases of being less severe and then more severe. For some people stress may be one of the driving factors behind this fluctuation.

The factors mentioned above as well as many others will now be elaborated on so that you can get a clearer picture of this strange disease.

The Development of Rheumatoid Arthritis

The development of rheumatoid arthritis does bear a few similarities to osteoarthritis. As with osteoarthritis, the mistake is often made that the symptoms become significant only in terms of treatment rather than as tools for diagnosis. This is far more detrimental in the case of rheumatoid arthritis, for three major reasons:

1 Rheumatoid arthritis can be considerably more severe than osteoarthritis, especially if the cause is not

addressed.
2 If sufferers assume they have a more common form of arthritis (such as osteoarthritis, rheumatism) and it turns out they have rheumatoid arthritis, the treatment will most likely have to change (effective treatments of the different forms can vary greatly).
3 Certain symptomatic treatments that are employed without consideration of the causes of rheumatoid arthritis may actually exacerbate these causes.

Clearly the bottom line is that if you choose to make the symptoms the main priority in rheumatoid arthritis, at least do not make them the *only* priority.

Now let us take a closer look at the common symptoms involved in this condition:

• Substantial swelling and inflammation of affected joints, beginning typically with the smaller joints and then spreading and leading to damage and eventual deformity
• Significant joint pain and stiffness
• Weakness, tiredness and a reduction of appetite
• Mild fever
• Possible association with non-joint tissues as well

INFLAMMATION
The discussion on inflammatory mechanisms in Chapter One applies even more to rheumatoid arthritis than to osteoarthritis. After all, the inflammation seen in rheumatoid arthritis is considerably more severe. Let us briefly review what processes may be causing this.

As you will recall, in osteoarthritis the occurrence of any inflammation is the result of various substances including histamine, leukotrienes and prostaglandins, among others. When the first stages of joint damage begin to occur, there is a release of inflammatory chemicals such as histamine from the mast cells. As histamine is released, which causes the increased permeability of the capillaries, local swelling results. Leukotrienes (produced in the body from oxidized polyunsaturated fatty acids) and certain prostaglandins (hormone-like substances from fats) are implicated as well. Leukotrienes are significantly involved in the healing process and inflammation in general, while certain prostaglandins (such as PGE2) account for general inflammation and increased temperature.

Although much more research needs to be done, there are some interesting correlations between inflammation in rheumatoid and osteoarthritis. It seems inconceivable that a condition such as osteoarthritis, which does such severe damage to the joints, would create less inflammation than other forms. Nevertheless, rheumatoid arthritis causes much greater inflammation. The reasons for this include:

- Osteoarthritis is generally fairly gradual in nature, thus producing less of an acute inflammatory reaction. Rheumatoid arthritis onset and subsequent development can be very fast and acute in comparison, thus leading to substantial inflammation (and also speeding up ancillary damage by lysosomal enzymes and cell-derived free radicals)
- Inflammatory responses are, to a great extent, mediated by the immune system. In rheumatoid arthritis, the immune system is often hyperactive and misfunctional
- Physical structure of the smaller joints allows for a more obvious appearance and sensation of swelling

The deleterious effect of the immune system (which will be explained shortly) spreads not only into the other joints but may also be associated with damage to other tissues such as the skin. Presumably, the tendency of the disease to spread to other joints is related to the body's auto-immunity to joint tissues in general. The spread to non-joint tissues may seem more difficult to explain. The truth is, while auto-immunity can be ascribed to a 'tissue-specific' misguidance of the immune system, it can also be caused by an immune system that is misguided in a more general manner. This may lead to significant problems, including other tissues being affected.

PAIN, STIFFNESS AND DEFORMITY

As well as accounting for much of the local swelling in the affected joints, histamine also activates 'pain fibres' in the area. The pain that is experienced can also be due to the subsequent joint damage. As in osteoarthritis, once the bones of the joint have been altered in their structure, this can lead to grinding of the bones and unavoidable irritation of local nerves.

The pain of rheumatoid arthritis can be quite constant and excruciating for some sufferers. We can draw some conclusions about this pain from the information we have on histamine and related inflammatory substances. In osteoarthritis, the local swelling is not nearly as acute. Thus we can assume that the release of inflammatory chemicals is not as much a factor in osteoarthritis; or because (in osteoarthritis) the release of these chemicals is spread out over a longer period of time, the pain caused is less intense. This leads us to the conclusion that a fair amount of the pain of osteoarthritis is attributable to the irritation of bone spurs (osteophytes) and the like.

Due to the extreme swelling that occurs with rheumatoid arthritis, we can also assume that the release of chemicals such as histamine, bradykinin, etc. is quite heavy. Because histamine and bradykinin are responsible for pain activation, and because joint deformity occurs in rheumatoid arthritis as well, these two chemicals have quite a severe influence on the physical discomfort of the condition.

The end result of rheumatoid arthritis, as far as the joint is concerned, is deformity. We have all seen the crooked and 'claw'-shaped hands of sufferers of various forms of arthritis. This is perhaps the classic example of the effects of the deformity. The integrity and shape of the joint can, of course, be significantly altered by the actual swelling itself, but this is not the end of the story. As you know, such joint damage generates certain processes; the three most significant ones involved in further destruction of the joint usually are:

1 Activation of lysosomal enzymes causes both the soft and hard tissue to be broken down.
2 White blood cell-derived free radicals (superoxides and peroxides) that are used for ridding the area of invaders such as bacteria inadvertently damage joint tissue.
3 Once the cartilage and synovial tissue are worn away by wear and by the two factors mentioned above the bones grind against one another, causing the ends to wear away. This eventually leads the body to repair the bone (albeit not in the intended shape of the original healthy joint).

This deformity can lead to loss of mobility. Although this is more common in the smallest joints such as those of the fingers and toes, varying degrees of immobility can occur in other joints as well.

FEVER AND FATIGUE

No doubt, many people are under the impression that the signs and symptoms of rheumatoid arthritis are limited to the joints. While it is true that the joints are initially the centre-point of the condition's manifestation, it is important to know that rheumatoid arthritis has an insidious habit of affecting other aspects of the body as well.

Prostaglandin E2 (PGE2) is greatly involved in rheumatoid arthritis, partly due to its role in the inflammatory process but also due to the fact that certain harmful micro-organisms may be involved (see below). The low-grade fever that can be experienced by many with rheumatoid arthritis may be linked to the activity of PGE2.

Earlier we looked at the role of prostaglandins in the general inflammatory process. Included in these effects was the elevation of body temperature. As you know, when you have an acute infection such as flu, you become feverish. This represents one of the body's defense mechanisms in eliminating the invading virus or bacteria. In the inflammatory process, the release of chemicals such as bradykinin or histamine results in local warmth. Besides their effect of increasing body temperature in general, prostaglandins augment the action of bradykinin and histamine.

The general fatigue that may be experienced can either be an indirect implication of the debilitating effects of rheumatoid arthritis – or perhaps something more specific. The truth is probably a combination of the two. One thing that comes to mind is the weakening effect of a constant hyperactivity of the immune system. Certain white blood cells, which are responsible for eliminating bacteria, viruses, cancer cells, debris, etc. need energy to work. In war, you would not expect a good performance out of the troops if you never fed them, would you? Your body allocates a great deal of energy to the white blood cells to help them to accomplish their tasks. Unfortunately this means that energy supplies may be drained more quickly. To make matters worse, these energy supplies are being used for what is generally an attack against one's own fortress!

Body Parts Affected

Before I go into an explanation of the immune system and mistaken identity, I will outline briefly once again the body parts affected by rheumatoid arthritis.

The actual nature of the joints affected by rheumatoid arthritis is, in the initial stages, less significant than in osteoarthritis. Although the joints in osteoarthritis require either significant wear and tear or perhaps chronic injury in order to become osteoarthritic, the same is not the case for rheumatoid arthritis. As mentioned, the trend is that the small joints are affected first, but if the condition persists it can spread to others. (*For more detailed information refer to Chapter One – the mechanics of the joint – and to the section earlier in this chapter (under 'Osteoarthritis') on the hands and knees*)

HANDS AND FEET

The joints in the hands and feet may not take as much obvious hammering as the weight-bearing joints of the hips, knees and spine, but they certainly do receive a huge amount of stress on a daily basis. The reason why certain joints are affected more than others may vary somewhat from person to person. Nevertheless, the severity of the condition in a particular joint may well be increased by any previous damage caused by wear and tear. The hands and feet are perfect examples of this; the fact that the finger and toe joints are smaller and have less protective tissue does not help.

KNEES, ANKLES, SHOULDERS, WRISTS AND ELBOWS

The knees and ankles are joints that certainly bear a great deal of weight on a day-to-day basis. They also are used very frequently. This adds up to a substantially higher susceptibility to damage in general. When you add the auto-immune effect to the equation, it is no wonder these joints are heavily damaged by rheumatoid arthritis. The shoulders, wrists and elbows are not weight-bearing, but they are used significantly and receive a great deal of stress.

These joints, as well as those of the fingers and toes, are all classed as synovial joints in that they have synovial membranes and the typical biochemistry that goes along with that designation (*see Chapter One for discussion on synovial joints*). The factors of lysosomal enzyme and free radical damage exist in rheumatoid arthritis as they do in osteoarthritis, although they are not as primary in the initial cause.

The Causes of Rheumatoid Arthritis

Rheumatoid arthritis is one of the most heavily studied of all health disorders, yet there are still major questions left unanswered as to how it occurs. The confusion stems in part from the fact that there may be several different reasons why it occurs, depending on the individual involved. We certainly know the end result of whatever is happening, and it is becoming ever clearer what causes the disease. What is a bit sketchy is what causes the cause. It is vital that still more research is done in this area to confirm what many experts believe triggers the cause. It is possible that the most scientifically accepted 'theories' on this dilemma are all correct – for certain cases. Other cases may be due to a combination of factors rather than just one. Fortunately, even though there is at least some lack of clarity on the 'causes of the cause', there appears to be ample scientific evidence on the basic 'why' of rheumatoid arthritis: auto-immunity.

AUTO-IMMUNITY

The whole idea of auto-immunity is not only quite fascinating but also could be seen as a bit bizarre and far-fetched. In spite of this, it is something that *does* exist, fortunately only in a minority of people. The medical and scientific community has included several different conditions in the category of 'auto-immune disorders'. Some of the more common and better known include:

• Rheumatoid arthritis
• Multiple sclerosis (MS)
• Systemic lupus erythematosus (SLE)
• Crohn's disease
• Juvenile-onset diabetes
• Ankylosing spondylitis
• Rheumatic fever

Some of these conditions are bound to be familiar to you. Many experts even consider that psoriasis may be linked with auto-immunity. As a matter of fact, there

are many connections between psoriasis and rheumatoid arthritis.

So what exactly is auto-immunity? As mentioned
earlier, auto-immunity is a strange but true phenome-
non wherein a person's immune system mistakenly
attacks normal tissues in the body. Perhaps now is a
good time to take a brief tour of the more basic parts
and functions of the immune system.

The Immune System

The immune system is among the most complex and
fascinating of all the functions of the human body. The
primary aim of the immune system is to protect the
body from disease and invasion from any harmful
substance. It also generally carries out the function of
making sure that *only what belongs* in the body enters or
remains in the body. This is a vital point to remember.

Now, from this information alone it is obvious that
this is an absolutely necessary process. If you did not
have a properly functioning immune system, you
would have no protection from harmful bacteria, viruses, cancer cells, or any other destructive force.

More than anything else, the immune system spends
its time patrolling the body looking for harmful bacteria, viruses and cancer cells to destroy. How it does
this is really quite remarkable. The complete process is
far too long and detailed to cover here, but we can look
at the most pertinent aspects of how this takes place.

The primary forces of the immune system are the
white blood cells. There are many different types of white
blood cells and each has its own specific mode of functioning. A few of the more pertinent cells are as follows:

- T-cells are derived from the thymus gland (behind the breastbone). They include *T-helper cells*, which encourage other white blood cells to attack and destroy invaders; *T-suppressor cells*, which, as you've probably guessed, discourage the attack and destruction of invaders by other white cells; and *cytotoxic T-cells*, which participate in the 'dirty work' and carry out destruction themselves. The T-helper and -suppressor cells are greatly responsible for mediating the activity of the immune system
- B-cells are white blood cells derived from the bone marrow. Their primary function is to make antibodies. Antibodies are proteins that carry out the more sophisticated function of the immune system: identifying invaders (refer to the section below on antibodies)
- Macrophages, neutrophils, and natural killer (NK) cells attack and destroy invading substances (such as bacteria, viruses, cancer cells and/or miscellaneous debris)

Antibodies

Without question, antibodies play the most important role in rheumatoid arthritis. Antibodies are proteins that are used to identify foreign invaders. Naturally, this is a very important piece to the immune puzzle. After all, if invaders are not identified, then they cannot be destroyed. Although certain other white blood cells can identify invaders, the majority of this process is carried out by the B-cell-derived antibodies.

The best way to explain antibodies is to use the example of immunization. For instance, when a child is vaccinated for small-pox, a very minute amount of small-pox is actually put into his or her body. At this point, the child's B-cells produce antibodies that actually match up to or bind to the small-pox. As part of this process the antibody will 'computerize' the identity of the small-pox, in a matter of speaking. The end result of this is that if small-pox ever enters the child again later in life, the 'small-pox antibodies' will recognize and bind to the new small-pox invader.

This process is fascinating enough in itself, but it is what happens next that finishes off the invader. You see, not only does an antibody identify invaders; it also starts an important chain reaction whereby they signal invader-destroying white blood cells to attack the substance. This communication and co-operation between antibodies and certain white blood cells is extremely valuable from the point of view of protecting us from the life-threatening potential of viruses, bacteria, and so on. Although this is only part of the functional capacity of the immune system, it should at least give you some idea of one of the most important processes relevant to rheumatoid arthritis.

Auto-immunity and Antibodies

All is fine when the antibodies and invader-destroying cells carry out their intended task fervently and efficiently. Imagine what would happen, however, if they were perhaps misinformed, misguided, or even out of control?

Where rheumatoid arthritis is concerned, something involving the immune system goes very, very wrong. The problem is not that the immune system components do not work, it is just that the wrong job is being done and/or in the wrong way. In rheumatoid arthritis the joint tissues are being attacked *in error* by the white blood cells. And what is signalling this attack? Typically it appears to be antibodies; antibodies which are supposed to be identifying invaders, not body parts! Calling it a case of mistaken identity may seem a bit of an understatement, but in rheumatoid arthritis this appears to be what happens.

What could possibly make the immune system attack the very body it is meant to protect? This is a compelling question that has a few possible answers depending on the person involved and his or her biological circumstances. While there are a handful of possible causes of auto-immunity in general, the following are the more likely factors in rheumatoid arthritis:

a Failure of the body's *self-identification system* to protect tissue cells from being attacked mistakenly
b Cross-reaction between normal body tissue antigen and an antibody at a point when an antibody binds to an invader;
c Damage to local tissue due to large-scale antigen–antibody activity in the area
d Weakened T-suppressor cell activity

In order to explain these possible reasons for auto-immunity properly, it is important to take a brief look at the body's *self-identification system*. It is undoubtedly one of the more interesting of the miracles of human biology.

Major Histocompatibility Complex (MHC) Antigens

Did you ever wonder why doctors have so much difficulty with organ transplants? After all, many techniques have been perfected that allow for great success in the actual surgery; yet there are still so many complications that can arise. No doubt you have heard of instances where the body of the person receiving the transplant 'rejects' the donor organ. This is where many of the complications begin.

You see, in the human body, essentially everything has been accounted for; a protective mechanism has been set up for almost any possibility. The immune system represents a major reason why the body stays how it is supposed to be and, as you may have guessed, it is the immune system that rejects the organ – *because the tissues of the transplanted organ are identified as being foreign*. But how does the body know? A heart is a heart; a kidney is a kidney – isn't it?

It is not the organ that is really rejected. It is the cells of the tissues of the organ that are considered invaders. How this works is that most cells in each person's body are marked with an 'identification tag' of sorts. Such a tag is called a *major histocompatibility complex (MHC) antigen* and it is attached to the surface of each cell. The term *antigen* refers to a substance of a particular chemical structure that is capable of being recognized by the immune system as being 'self' or 'non-self' (in other words either belonging in the body or not belonging in the body). MHC antigens signify 'self', or those that belong. These special MHC identification tags are much like fingerprints in that they are unique to each individual. Identical twins actually have MHCs in common with one another, but the further removed one is from another, genetically speaking, the less likely is the sharing of common MHCs.

Considering this information on MHCs, it becomes much easier to understand how the immune system identifies and differentiates foreign invaders from 'self'. In many cases, this is the basis of auto-immunity. It certainly does not take a stretch of the imagination to see how auto-immunity could be negatively influenced by a fault in this 'self'/'non-self' system. In a war, for instance, each side will need to have some method of differentiating itself from the enemy. This keeps each side from attacking the wrong people. The same thing is true in the body. One could call the MHC a sort of emblem showing that a cell is 'one of us'.

All things seem possible in the body, including failures. Technically speaking, a failure could occur whereby the self-identification system fails in the cells of a particular tissue. In principle, this would probably be more likely to occur in tissue cells that have already been damaged or mutated, perhaps by free radicals or certain toxins.

The second auto-immunity scenario is perhaps a bit less clear cut. As you know, antibodies attach themselves to invaders, which they identify. This initiates the destruction of the invader by certain white blood cells. The antibody also computerizes the identity of that particular invader and will automatically attach to, and signal the destruction of, the same substance at any point in the future. This works well, *unless* a tissue cell antigen is similar to an invading antigen at the time of the computerization of the identity of the invader.

If this happens, antibodies induced to an invader may also erroneously *cross-react* with *normal tissue antigens* and computerize their identity! As you can guess, this would lead to a habitual destruction of all joint tissue cells bearing the same identity tag as those tissue cells that were wrongly identified in the first place. This explains why auto-immune diseases are typically degenerative in nature. It may also explain why rheumatoid arthritis progresses in a symmetrical manner. In other words, if the tissues of one hand are 'identified' wrongly as a non-self antigen, then presumably the other hand would be identified this way as well, due to common tissue characteristics.

Although there is no unanimous consensus on what causes this cross-reaction to occur, evidence seems to point to bacteria or food antigens as being likely instigators.

Even if there is no cross-reaction due to misidentification, normal tissue antigens can still be adversely affected. This third scenario is probably best explained by analogy. For instance, in any battle not only are the intended targets (such as buildings, people, tanks, etc.) damaged by bombs and bullets; the actual ground underneath and around the target is destroyed as well. When a battle between white blood cells occurs in or around joint tissues, the surrounding tissue can be injured in the process.

In one common situation, the invader-destroying white blood cells use some nasty toxin (such as superoxide radicals) to kill the invader. As you may recall, superoxides and related free radicals also damage joint tissue.

Another situation where injury to surrounding tissue occurs relates to the existence of antigen–antibody complexes. Simply put, tissue irritation and eventual injury can take place when a complex of an antibody bound to an antigen remains in the tissues for a long time before being 'cleaned up' by debris-collecting white cells.

The fourth possibility relates to the immune-regulating mechanism of the T-suppressor cells. The T-suppressor cells are the thymus-derived white blood cells that are responsible for discouraging excessive activity of other white blood cells involved in the destruction of invaders. There are two ways in which a T-suppressor cell dysfunction can encourage auto-immunity.

As you might expect, the body has defense mechanisms against improper or overactive cellular functioning. The T-suppressor cells serve this purpose where the immune system is concerned. If T-suppressor cells are malfunctioning (as any cell is capable of doing at a given time) then any inappropriate or over-zealous antibody responses may not be controlled.

There are occasions when a person's suppressor cells are able to function properly but the thymus is producing too few in proportion to the T-helper cells. This situation appears to be particularly common in food allergy sufferers. This will be discussed in more detail below.

Whether a person's auto-immune reaction is produced due to improper identification, cross-reaction, peripheral damage or suppressor cell problems, the bottom line is that the joints may well become an undeserving target of attack. Methods of possibly reducing auto-immunity will be covered in Chapter Four.

Food Allergies

It may seem a bit strange that the issue of food allergies would be brought up in a discussion of rheumatoid arthritis, but there does appear to be a link in some sufferers. Without going into too much detail, food allergies may cause or exacerbate rheumatoid arthritis tendencies in a few different ways.

It would appear that the more non-self antigens that are floating through the bloodstream, the more likely it is that an auto-immune reaction will occur. After all, this would make the immune system 'hyper-alert', so to speak, and this would be likely to lead to immune hyperactivity. The more antibodies and destroyer cells patrolling the system, the greater the chance of:

a Accidental attack of 'self' tissue antigens

b Peripheral damage to tissues in the surrounding area
   of an immune attack
c Injury to the tissues from antigen–antibody complexes

Food components that are not intended to be
absorbed into the bloodstream intact represent a plentiful source of non-self antigens. Proteins that are not
digested completely into their component parts (free
amino acids) are the most likely culprits. Any similarity
between a food protein antigen and a tissue antigen
may cause misidentification and/or cross-reaction to
occur. Also, the more food antigens in the blood and
tissues, the more likely the above problems are to arise.
This may help explain why research has verified a
significant improvement in many rheumatoid arthritis
sufferers who have eliminated foods to which they
turned out to be allergic.

(For more information on food allergies and their
treatment, it is suggested you consult the book *Allergies*
in this series.)

It should now be clear that rheumatoid arthritis is a
potentially serious and complicated condition. This is
especially true due to the insidious and often
unchecked attack of one's own body by the immune
system. Remember, the memory of antibodies is
designed to be permanent.

Prompt diagnosis and action are urgently recommended. Regardless of exactly what your arthritis is
caused by, it is of vital importance to know which type
you have. This is particularly true of rheumatoid arthritis, because special testing procedures may be necessary in order to confirm a diagnosis. Once a diagnosis is
made, treatment and prevention of further destruction
are of prime importance. In Chapter Four we will look

at many of the methods which have been found to be of value in treating and/or preventing those factors involved in rheumatoid arthritis. These methods utilize medically and scientifically researched vitamins, minerals, herbs and other natural substances as well as dietary changes.

OTHER COMMON ARTHRITIS-RELATED PROBLEMS

Although osteo- and rheumatoid arthritis get a lot of the attention where arthritis is concerned, there are many other related conditions that can be quite prevalent. They may not always be as complicated or as ultimately destructive as rheumatoid or osteoarthritis, but they are aggravating and potentially debilitating none the less.

Many of the other forms of arthritis fall under the very general headings of either *rheumatism*, *arthralgia*, or perhaps just plain *arthritis*. There are far too many to discuss here, but we will look very briefly at a few of the more common arthritis-related problems.

Rheumatism is a term which is frequently used to categorize several conditions. It is far from being a specific classification and is perhaps the most general and all-encompassing of all the categories related to arthritis. The basic definition of rheumatism includes those disorders associated with joint and/or muscle pain and stiffness. Arthralgia refers to conditions involving general joint pain. As we have discussed, the term arthritis basically means 'inflammation of the joint'. Although we have seen the potential problems of not having a more specific diagnosis, at least there are some general approaches that may be of value for arthritis conditions other than osteo- and rheumatoid arthritis.

Certain forms of arthritis may be caused by factors quite apart from the actual joints themselves. For instance, when we look at rheumatoid arthritis we see the influence of the bone marrow (B-cells, antibodies) and the thymus gland (T-cells); perhaps genetic factors may be involved; dietary and lifestyle issues need to be taken into consideration; and so on. Osteoarthritis brings factors other than the joints into the equation as well, such as age, sex, diet and lifestyle, etc. On the other hand, there are several arthritic disorders that are greatly dependent on factors specific to the joints. Conditions such as *bursitis, tendonitis*, sports injuries and repetitive strain injuries seem to be more centred on the specific location affected. They also tend not to spread in the same manner as both rheumatoid and osteoarthritis can. Having said this, *every* different form of arthritis and/or rheumatism can be influenced, either before or after the fact, by diet and lifestyle.

Bursitis

Bursitis is a form of arthritis that involves inflammation of the *bursa*. As you may remember, the bursa is a small membrane found in certain joint areas which carries out functions similar to those of a synovial membrane, including providing lubricating fluid for easier mobility of the joint. Areas that are frequently affected by this type of inflammation include, among others, the elbows, shoulders and knees.

Bursitis can be an eventual complication of an existing arthritic problem afflicting a joint. The probability increases as the joint space becomes more and more damaged and narrowed. Also, the destructive effects of lysosomal enzymes can certainly damage the bursa. This points to the breakdown of neighbouring synovial tissue as being a likely factor.

Another common cause of bursitis is either repeated or extreme pressure or trauma. For example, many athletes develop such problems due either to a consistent strain or repeated movements that test the limits of how the joint is mechanically supposed to move. The trauma does not have to be repeated, though. If there is a severe stress injury to a particular joint, this can start the unfortunate process as well.

When a joint is damaged, either by bursitis itself or by another form of arthritis, tiny spurs or deposits of bone-like material can develop in the area of the bursa as a result of the joint's (often faulty) attempts at repair. This will increase the pain as well as reducing the chances of eliminating the bursitis.

Tendonitis

The tendons are strong yet flexible tissue that attach muscles to bones. They have a 'band-like' characteristic and can usually withstand the ordinary strains applied to them by muscle and surrounding joint movement. However, as you might expect, if there is repeated excessive strain or a severe injury that tests the tendon's limits past a certain point, tendonitis can develop.

The inflammation and pain involved in tendonitis are quite aggravating and naturally they can significantly reduce a person's ability (and willingness) to move the muscles or joints in the surrounding area. The heel (Achilles tendon) is one of the better-known areas affected by tendonitis, but the shoulders, knees, elbows and others are also prone to this problem. As in bursitis, bony deposits can develop in the tendon areas thereby causing extra pain and making the condition more difficult to get rid of.

Sports Injuries and Arthritis

Sports injuries represent one of the more common causes of osteoarthritis, bursitis and tendonitis, especially in younger people. Where osteoarthritis is concerned, we know that wear and tear plays a major role in its development. If wear and tear is accelerated by injury, age becomes less of a factor.

'Tennis elbow' may be one of the more well-known arthritic problems related to sports injuries, but literally any mobile joint can be affected. The body is just *not* designed to withstand and compensate for some of the more extreme actions that regularly occur in various sports. When you look at contact sports such as rugby or American football, the participants often have to go to extremes to build up a greater volume of surrounding muscle tissue, in part to support the tenuous integrity of the threatened joints. The same thing is true to a lesser extent of other sports that heavily tax the joints.

While athletes are prime candidates for bursitis and tendonitis, these conditions can afflict anyone. Under optimal circumstances, both of these disorders should clear up reasonably well over a matter of days or weeks with appropriate rest. There are, however, factors that will reduce the chances of a quick or proper healing process:

- If the affected area is not rested
- If the neighbouring joint(s) is/are significantly damaged by arthritis in general
- If dietary and lifestyle factors exacerbate the condition

Bursitis, tendonitis and general sports and repeated

strain injuries have some similar dynamics, even though they might affect different tissues. The effective ways of dealing with their treatment, symptomatically and otherwise, tends to be somewhat similar as well. This will be discussed in Chapter Four.

When discussing any health disorder that involves pain, damage to necessary body functions and degeneration, it is difficult not to become quite aggravated and depressed by it. The development and progression of conditions such as rheumatoid and osteoarthritis seem so forceful and predetermined that sufferers often feel quite impotent to do anything but ease the agony temporarily. This is a terrible state for anyone to be in and may cause sufferers to give up and accept that they will be in ever-increasing misery.

It must be said again that this attitude of helplessness is, if anything, perpetuated by the heavy marketing of over-the-counter pain relievers such as aspirin, paracetamol and ibuprofen. While these medications can serve to reduce pain and inflammation for a while, they also have a negative side that you rarely hear about.

It may not have to be this way for those suffering with even the most debilitating arthritic conditions. As a matter of fact, there is a great deal of published medical and scientific research that *proves* that there is much that can be done to:

1 Treat the symptoms of arthritis *without* drugs and with almost no risk of side-effects
2 Correct many of the factors that may cause or perpetuate arthritis development
3 Help prevent arthritis development in the first place

Why this valuable information is not given to arthritis

sufferers more frequently is anybody's guess, but the intention of this book is to set the record straight and provide sufferers with the tools to gain control over their arthritis – once and for all. Such information on arthritis treatment can be found in Chapter Four; first, in the next chapter, we will examine some of the orthodox medical treatments available.

CHAPTER 3

Common Medical Treatments for Arthritis

There is no question that the debilitating nature of arthritis and its prevalence have prompted great emphasis on its treatment over the years. This is quite fortunate, but from the point of view of drug therapy, the medical community has had only a limited scope with which to deal with the problem. This is especially true of the most degenerative forms such as rheumatoid and osteoarthritis. Why is this the case, when so much time, effort and money have presumably been channelled into research?

First of all, in order to be successful in treating a condition, one must address all its angles. This would include arresting the condition's development by addressing its cause, relieving the symptoms and, if possible, preventing it from recurring or even from occurring in the first place.

Now, preventing arthritis may never be within the remit of standard drug therapy. (Fortunately there are plenty of non-drug methods which may offer great promise – *see Chapter Four*.) When it comes to its cause, or arresting its development, the availability and success of drugs depends on what type of arthritis one is dealing with. The truth is, even if such drugs are available, as in the case of rheumatoid arthritis, the benefits are limited and the risks and possible side-effects are vast and severe. Where symptoms are concerned there is no lack of medication regardless of the type of arthritis, but the benefits are far from perfect and the risks go deeper than just the obvious side-effects.

The bottom line is that, in spite of any possible benefits, drugs for arthritis do not create fewer sufferers, they do not cure arthritis, and they can have their own damaging consequences. In order to weigh the possible benefits against the risks, it is important to know the background of a few of the more common standard drug therapies used.

PLEASE NOTE: In spite of what you learn in this chapter, it is essential that you do *not* discontinue any *prescribed* drugs without consulting a doctor first. Good or bad, many drugs can create a dependence to varying degrees and discontinuing their use too quickly may have negative consequences. Do *not* take this warning lightly. It is not just a formality!

NON-STEROIDAL ANTI-INFLAMMATORY DRUGS (NSAIDS)

The category of drugs called non-steroidal anti-inflammatory drugs (NSAIDs) represents the most common type of medication used in arthritis treatment. NSAIDs can be useful for many sufferers in the temporary relief of pain, swelling, heat and redness, but not everyone will benefit from their use in the same way. It is generally recommended that if they have not worked for the pain within a week or so, and if they do not help the swelling within a few weeks, they are not likely to be of value. Still, as a rule, temporary reduction of some of the symptoms is likely to occur.

The more well-known NSAIDs include:

- Aspirin
- Ibuprofen
- Indomethacin
- Naproxen
- Fenoprofen

Each different NSAID has its own specific characteristics, but their effects are usually quite similar, at least as far as pain and inflammation are concerned. The more common side-effects of each are often similar as well.

How They Work

As you know, NSAIDs can be of some benefit in arthritis due to their ability to reduce pain and the symptoms of inflammation such as swelling, heat and redness in the affected joints. In order to understand the way they accomplish this, we must go back to how certain chemicals cause inflammation in the first place.

As you will recall, *prostaglandins* are the hormone-like substances derived from fats which mediate inflammation, pain and body temperature. Prostaglandin E2 (PGE2) is the primary prostaglandin involved in *inducing* pain and inflammation. PGE2 becomes active in arthritis as a result of joint tissue damage, and it augments the effects of inflammatory chemicals such as bradykinin and histamine.

From this context you may already be able get some idea of how NSAIDs work to fight the symptoms of arthritis. NSAIDs basically block the production of inflammatory prostaglandins, thereby reducing PGE2 levels. This in turn leads to reduced inflammation, pain and, if applicable, fever – at least temporarily.

The way in which NSAIDs work may sound like the answer to an arthritis sufferer's prayer. However, while there can at times be considerable temporary relief, there is a negative side to NSAIDs which must be understood. Of course, many NSAIDs are well known, popular and are available over the counter. This tends to encourage their frequent use without the advice of a doctor. Unfortunately, this may also lead inadvertently to people not addressing the possible side-effects and contra-indications (that is, those circumstances under which these drugs should *not* be used), nor following the appropriate dosage requirements and general precautions.

Potential Side-effects and Contra-indications

The possible side-effects and contra-indications of NSAIDs may vary somewhat depending on the particular drug being considered, but some general concerns do exist. Possible side-effects include:

- Stomach or intestinal irritation
- Stomach or intestinal ulcers
- Tinnitus (ringing in the ears)
- Reduced blood-clotting ability
- Allergic reaction such as asthma
- Dizziness
- Blurred vision
- Liver damage (very rare)
- Kidney damage (very rare)

NSAIDs should *not* be used when a person is:

- Pregnant or breastfeeding

- Allergic to aspirin or other NSAIDs
- Taking other anti-coagulant drugs (unless advised by doctor)

Nor should they be used when a person has:

- A history of or current stomach or intestinal ulcers
- A history of or current liver or kidney disease
- A history or current heart disorders (unless advised by a doctor)
- Haemophilia or other blood-clotting disorders

There is another major side-effect which is very seldom reported but which has been proven in published research. This research was particularly relevant to osteoarthritis but would presumably apply to any chronic form of arthritis. The research has shown that NSAIDs actually *reduce* the ability of cartilage to be repaired and *increase* the speed of cartilage destruction in osteoarthritis! This is probably due to an adverse effect on the body's general ability to manufacture the collagen and/or related matrix materials found in cartilage. This disturbing data was published in world-renowned medical journals such as *The Lancet* and *Journal of Rheumatology*. Considering the fact that NSAIDs represent the first and the most common treatment of osteoarthritis and probably of most other forms of arthritis, only one conclusion can be drawn: NSAIDs may well perpetuate and worsen the very arthritis they are being used to treat. Remember, cartilage destruction can be an eventual outcome of both osteo- *and* rheumatoid arthritis, so we should not assume that NSAIDs affect only *osteo*arthritis adversely.

Unfortunately, this is not the only example of a class

of drugs that provides a beneficial symptomatic effect which masks an insidious degenerative effect on the same condition.

When we look at how NSAIDs work (by blocking prostaglandins) another concern creeps in. NSAIDs do not only block prostaglandin E2; they block prostaglandins in general. PGE1, PGE2 and other prostaglandins are needed in order for many necessary bodily processes to occur, and any indiscriminate blocking of their activity can be damaging to the body in ways too numerous to elaborate here.

Presumably, the moral of this story should be:

a Unless *prescribed* continually, NSAIDs should only be used as seldom as possible and for as short a time as possible
b There may be side-effects of over-the-counter medication which will not appear on the label

STEROIDAL ANTI-INFLAMMATORY DRUGS (CORTICOSTEROIDS)

The class of drugs called steroidal anti-inflammatory drugs or *corticosteroids* are not used in all forms of arthritis; generally they are employed for only a relatively small selection of health disorders, such as:

• Some cases of rheumatoid arthritis
• Certain other auto-immune conditions (such as systemic lupus erythematosus)
• Severe allergic reactions (such as asthma)
• Ulcerative inflammatory bowel disease (Crohn's disease)
• Various skin conditions (such as eczema and psoriasis)

The body actually produces corticosteroids (often called 'steroids' for short) and related hormones in the adrenal glands. Among other things, the hormones of the adrenal glands (such as adrenaline and cortisone) mediate the body's reactions to stress, suppress inflammatory responses, suppress immune responses and carry out several different metabolic functions.

As you might expect, corticosteroid drugs have much the same basic properties as the hormones produced naturally in the body. The main purposes for which corticosteroid drugs are used include:

• Anti-inflammatory action
• Immune suppression
• Anti-allergic action

There are many different biological effects of corticosteroid drugs on the human body, but very few of them are positive. The reason that we derive benefit from the corticosteroids made by the body is that their levels are mediated and controlled by the body's requirements and circumstances. However, when they are introduced to the body from outside, the levels are not being controlled, dictated and released with respect to the body's moment-to-moment requirements. Because of the extremely profound effects of such hormones on body processes, excessive amounts can cause severe harm.

In rheumatoid arthritis, corticosteroids may be used because of their anti-inflammatory and immune suppressive effects. The anti-inflammatory activity of corticosteroids bears some similarity to that of the non-steroidal anti-inflammatory drugs, in that they block prostaglandin production. Corticosteroids suppress immunity by reducing the activity of both T-cells and antibody-producing B-cells. The temporary suppression of the misguided attack on the joint by white blood cells may reduce or halt the progression of the damage, but this benefit lasts for only a limited period of time. It is temporary not so much because the corticosteroids are less effective over time, but because they are too harmful to be taken in large amounts over extended periods of time. This is one of the main reasons why these drugs are not used more universally. It is also why the medical community is testing other drugs that have immuno-suppressive effects without so many other damaging metabolic effects.

CORTICOSTEROIDS: POSSIBLE SIDE-EFFECTS
- Fluid retention
- Weight gain
- Increased blood sugar (can be very severe)
- Bone loss (increasing risk of osteoporosis)
- Weakened immunity to infection
- 'Moon face' (altered shape of the lower part of face)
- Mood swings
- Menstrual problems
- Impotence
- High blood pressure (at times severe)
- Thinning of the skin
- Fat deposits in the face and upper back
- Muscle wasting
- Depression (sometimes very severe)
- Nervousness
- Insomnia
- Damage to adrenal glands (thereby reducing the body's own ability to produce its own adrenal hormones)

- Damage to the thymus gland

Considering the duration and serious nature of many of the side-effects, it is no wonder many medical books and medical doctors warn of the dangers of corticosteroids and encourage all efforts to find a safer alternative to provide the necessary results. In particular, the increased blood sugar and blood pressure, weakened immunity and bone loss can be quite dangerous and it is imperative for the possible benefits to be weighed against these considerable risks. It would appear that many in the medical community are taking this into consideration of their own accord, but it is always vitally important for the *patient* also to be aware of any risks associated with a prescribed or over-the-counter drug.

Due to the risks, the medical community has tried to use local application whenever possible, but this certainly does not eliminate all the risks as absorption into the bloodstream still takes place. In cases where rheumatoid arthritis has spread throughout the body, using a local injection becomes, in any event, less practical.

OTHER ANTI-RHEUMATIC DRUGS

Although non-steroidal anti-inflammatory drugs are generally the first type of drug employed for most forms of arthritis, with rheumatoid arthritis the treatment generally becomes much more aggressive as the disease worsens. Corticosteroids are used in many severe cases, but often they are avoided for as long as possible in favour of drugs such as *gold*, *chloroquine*, or *penicillamine*.

These drugs are quite potent and potentially quite dangerous; however, on occasion they seem to reduce the progression of the joint destruction. In order to achieve this goal using these drugs, however, frequently they must be taken for long periods of time. As you might expect, treatment in these circumstances is often abandoned due to the ever increasing risks and toxicity to the body. The problem here stems from the fact that these drugs act more slowly than other arthritis treatments and, of course, they are very toxic.

The exact actions of these drugs has been analysed, but there still seems to be a less than perfect understanding of their mechanism in slowing the progression of rheumatoid arthritis. Gold, either by injection or taken orally, seems to reduce the production of white blood cells by the bone marrow. Because such bone marrow-derived cells make antibodies, presumably this reduction in their numbers reduces the antibody-binding and subsequent attack of the joint tissues. Unfortunately, not only would this impair *necessary* immune function, but gold can also be toxic to the kidneys and blood.

Chloroquine is actually an anti-malarial drug that just happens to have an application in rheumatoid arthritis. It is also very toxic. Vision damage is a common risk when high doses of this drug are used. Headaches, nausea, convulsions, rashes and many other problems are also possible.

Penicillamine (no relation to the antibiotic penicillin) is often used as an alternative to gold. Allergic reactions are not unusual, however, and kidney and blood damage are constantly having to be checked for. Nausea, mouth ulcers and a loss of the sense of taste are among a long list of other possible side-effects.

External Preparations
External preparations, often called *rheumatic rubs*, can

offer some temporary symptomatic relief when applied locally. Ointments, cremes, lotions, etc. used for this purpose may contain substances such as camphor or methyl salicylate. They can be used without too many concerns by most sufferers, but allergic skin reactions can occur. It is also important to avoid applying them to too large a surface area, and to avoid broken or irritated skin as well as the areas around the eyes and nose. They are also not recommended for children.

As you can see, there are quite severe limitations to the value of NSAIDs, corticosteroids and other anti-rheumatic drugs used in the treatment of rheumatoid arthritis. In spite of the fact that they can actually serve a therapeutic purpose (although their success rate is far from 100 per cent), it must be considered thoroughly whether the benefits outweigh the risks. It would appear that *this* is where these drugs often fall flat.

WARNING: If you are currently being *prescribed* any drug for the treatment of any form of arthritis, do not discontinue the drug(s) without first consulting your doctor (and preferably the acting specialist). Many such drugs can cause severe problems if eliminated too quickly. Take this warning very seriously!

CHAPTER 4

Natural Treatment of Arthritis

PART 1: FOODS AND ARTHRITIS

After such a depressing and gloomy look at the common medical drugs used to treat arthritis, we could not be blamed for feeling that there is little we can do to fight the progressive worsening of arthritis. It is true that the severe limitations of these drugs do *not* only relate to their obvious side-effects. We also have to consider the dubious value of even the safest of the common arthritis drugs, the NSAIDs. There is no question that even *temporary* pain relief is valuable to any arthritis sufferer, but when we look at the proven destructive effect of NSAIDs on the cartilage, it cannot help but take off much of their gloss, so to speak.

The good news is, in spite of the limitations and risks of arthritis drugs, there is *proven medical benefit* to many methods of treating arthritis naturally – *without the high risk of side-effects or contra-indications*.

It is unfortunate that the orthodox medical approach to most any health disorder manages to take control *away* from the patient as much as possible, rather than to *give* the patient as much control as possible. It must be said that there is perhaps a significant emotional, mental and maybe even therapeutic value in being able to take a hand in your own treatment. If such a thing were possible (which it most definitely is in this case) this would also help to obliterate much of the helplessness and desperation that may accompany such a debilitating and degenerative disorder.

Undoubtedly you have heard the phrase, 'It's not always what you *do* do that counts – sometimes it's what you *don't* do.' Well, to a certain extent this adage applies to the issue of arthritis control, at least from the standpoint of diet. Our diet influences every aspect of our bodies on a day-to-day basis. This is true from both a positive and negative standpoint. In other words, if we eat the right things, we can expect to be more healthy overall; if we eat the wrong things, we can expect to be less healthy. This is probably understood even by those who are not the slightest bit concerned about proper dietary habits. After all, many of us heard it from our parents from the very beginning!

The problem is, 'healthy' is such a general term that it has little meaning for many people. People may not actually equate 'healthy' with 'free from disease or illness'. While no diet can promise guaranteed freedom from disease or illness, medical and scientific research have confirmed that dietary manipulation may have a significant effect on the progression of arthritis in general – on both its symptoms and on factors involved in its cause and/or development.

Fats

From the standpoint of arthritis, the role of dietary fats cannot be overstated. In our society we have the impression of fats being something we like but should not eat. If we choose a lifestyle that adopts a 'self-discipline stance', then we are prone to bend over backwards to avoid *all* fats. (Some people may classify this as a 'self-*torture* stance'!) Whether you think this is a prudent step toward better health or an exercise in dietary masochism, such judgements should not be made without having all the facts. Besides which, many people have formulated an opinion on the fat issue on the basis of looks rather than true inner health.

There is nothing wrong with disciplining yourself in order to look better, but would you still adopt such an approach at the expense of your health? This is where the confusion lies. We are being influenced in such a way that we have little choice but to assume that eating fat, in general, is bad. Is this really true? Well, it depends entirely on what *type* of fat you are talking about.

ANIMAL FATS VS VEGETABLE FATS

Fats are found in a large proportion of the foods we eat each day. Sometimes the fat is naturally occurring in the food in certain amounts; often it is added to a food during the processing methods. Many people are aware of the difference between saturated or unsaturated fats, or perhaps between animal or vegetable fats. While these are important issues to health in general, there are other factors that may be even more relevant to arthritis. The following is a list of some of the more common foods that contain fats:

- Dairy products
- Meats (such as beef, pork, lamb)
- Poultry
- Eggs
- Fish
- Vegetable oils

- Seeds
- Whole grains
- Beans (such as soybeans)

Animal products are bound to contain higher amounts of saturated fats. Foods such as fatty fish, seeds, whole grains, nuts and beans contain good amounts of unsaturated fats (especially of the polyunsaturated variety). An easy way to tell the difference is that saturated fats become solid at room temperature, while unsaturated fats remain liquid.

Fats are broken down in the body into what are known as *fatty acids*. Your body actually needs certain fatty acids (called *essential fatty acids*) in order to make substances that are necessary to its function. You could not live without an adequate supply of the essential fatty acids, which are *linoleic acid* and *linolenic acid*.

So exactly what do fats have to do with arthritis?

INFLAMMATORY PROSTAGLANDINS AND LEUKOTRIENES

As mentioned in Chapter One, the hormone-like substances called prostaglandins are manufactured from unsaturated fats. There are different prostaglandins and they carry out different essential functions such as controlling blood-clotting and, of course, mediating inflammation. The different types of prostaglandins are categorized in series. The ones most relevant to the subject of arthritis are:

1 Prostaglandin 1 series
2 Prostaglandin 2 series (which includes PGE2)
3 Prostaglandin 3 series

As you know, PGE2 is manufactured from arachidonic acid (derived from animal fat). Although PGE2 can be made *in smaller but adequate quantities* from non-animal sources, animal fats can elevate PGE2 to *excessive* levels quickly and significantly. This effect can be quite disastrous in arthritis, as PGE2 triggers inflammation. The local swelling, pain and heat of arthritis can definitely be linked to increased levels of inflammatory prostaglandins in the affected joints and, besides this, inflammatory prostaglandins also augment the inflammatory effects of histamine and histamine-like chemicals.

Nor do the problems brought on by excessive PGE2 stop there. You then have to worry about the prostaglandin-induced inflammation initiating lysosomal enzyme damage. You do not need to be reminded of the problems this can lead to!

Leukotrienes have also been discussed in Chapter One. The most inflammatory leukotrienes, which can be hundreds of times more inflammatory than histamine, are also derived from arachidonic acid metabolism. The healing benefits and the inflammatory mechanism of leukotrienes can be of value in the earlier stages of joint damage; however, over the long term they enhance the processes leading to lysosomal enzyme damage and, as such, they quickly wear out their welcome.

Whether looking at inflammatory symptoms or the subsequent joint destruction caused by inflammation, the conclusion is very clear: the excessive intake of arachidonic acid should be avoided if you suffer with arthritis!

Just as a reminder, the main foods that contain arachidonic acid include, among others: beef, pork, lamb, dairy products (milk, cheese, etc.), poultry, etc.

Once again, if you have arthritis, especially a degenerative form such as rheumatoid or osteoarthritis, you should seriously consider reducing significantly or even eliminating these foods from your diet, at least temporarily, due to their enhancement of inflammatory prostaglandin and leukotriene levels.

UNSATURATED FATS AND PEROXIDATION

As if the role of *animal* fats were not bad enough, there is also a problem with *non*-animal fats *used in cooking*. The trend towards using vegetable oils over animal fats has been encouraging, if somewhat misplaced. You see, unsaturated fats have many wonderful attributes from a health standpoint. They are healthier to the cardiovascular system, they are anti-inflammatory, they are important for proper immune function, and so on – *but only when consumed uncooked!* The problem is, the value of unsaturated fats is entirely dependent on the fats maintaining their intended chemical characteristics. You do not have to be a chemist to appreciate this point. After all, a racing car would not be nearly as valuable nor effective if someone sneaked into the garage and put a domestic car's engine in it!

All fats have their own molecular structure. Unfortunately, unsaturated fats have a structure that is quite susceptible to alteration or damage. It is oxygen that *oxidizes* unsaturated fats. This oxidation process is speeded up significantly by heat, causing the fat to become *peroxidized*. Of course, peroxides are one of the most destructive free radicals to the joints. The higher the heat and the longer the exposure, the more peroxidation occurs – and thus, the more damage caused to the joints. As a result, fried foods, cooked oils in general, barbecued and flame-grilled meats and any other source of fat that has been heated (especially at high temperatures) should be avoided.

Hydrogenated and *partially hydrogenated fats*, such as those found in standard margarines and many other food products (read labels) are some of the most inflammatory, cardiovascular-damaging and free radical-producing foods that exist. Hydrogenated fats have been intentionally altered, molecularly speaking, and heated to absurd temperatures all in the interest of creating a solid vegetable fat with a longer shelf life. If only the makers had taken into consideration *your* shelf life! Needless to say, hydrogenated and partially hydrogenated fats should be significantly reduced or eliminated from the diet of any arthritis sufferer.

Avoiding animal fats is clearly an important goal in arthritis, but so is the elimination of vegetable fats that have been cooked at high temperature (e.g. fried) or are hydrogenated. Feel free to consume *raw* vegetable oils, provided they are fresh and unrefined.

ANTI-INFLAMMATORY FATS

We have certainly and deservedly raked arachidonic acid over the coals, and we already know that heated or hydrogenated fats can be quite harmful. We have also discussed the fact that vegetable oils may be of value provided they are raw and fresh. The use of certain types of non-vegetable dietary fats can actually have a beneficial effect as well. The dietary sources of non-vegetable fats that may provide a benefit in arthritis include, among others, oil from fatty fish such as:

- Salmon
- Mackerel
- Herring
- Cod

These fish can be quite valuable provided that they are not cooked improperly. Poaching or steaming them is perhaps the best way to get the benefit without damaging the fats they contain.

In order to understand why these fish may be so helpful when other non-vegetable oils are so harmful, we must look back to the other prostaglandin series that we have yet to discuss – series PG1 and PG3. The type of fatty acids contained in such fish belong to the PG3 series. These fish contain fatty acids such as *EPA* (eicosapentaenoic acid) and *DHA* (docosahexaenoic acid). These are classed as *omega 3 fatty acids*. EPA, in particular, will be discussed in more depth in Part Two of this chapter, but suffice it to say that the PG3 series is useful in arthritis mostly because it has significant *anti*-inflammatory activity.

It is clear that fats play perhaps the biggest role, in terms of diet, in the development of arthritis, not only as regards symptoms (inflammation) but also the disease's progression (free radicals, inflammation leading to lysosomal enzyme damage). As you will find out later in this chapter, fats can even play a role in either encouraging or discouraging auto-immunity. Regardless of what type of arthritis you have, eliminating or reducing all animal fat and heated or hydrogenated vegetable oils is highly recommended.

Sugar

Sugar is another one of those 'foods' that we know or think we know we should not eat. Sugar represents a source of many of today's most damaging health problems, yet it is needed by every cell of the body in order to live.

All sugar is broken down and used or is stored until it is converted into usable blood sugar (glucose). The storage capacity of sugar in the body is not always manifested in a desirable way. For instance, if an abundance of sugar is entering the system on a regular basis *before* the stored sugar is used up, any excess that is not needed immediately can be stored – *as fat*. We already know that obesity is only going to put more strain on the joints, especially in osteoarthritis, but this is not even the main concern.

The consumption of sugar causes a release of the adrenal hormone called adrenaline. Among other functions, adrenaline, like corticosteroids, has the ability to reduce inflammation. Now, on the surface this may sound like a great reason to eat sugar by the bucketful if you have arthritis, but nothing could be further from the truth! Why? Well, we do not have a 'bottomless pit' of adrenaline. The problem with indiscriminately stimulating the release of adrenaline is that at a certain point the excessive release begins to exhaust the supply. If sugar is consumed too regularly, the constant release of adrenaline may also cause the adrenal glands to become sluggish. This would mean that they would work less efficiently in releasing both adrenaline *and* corticosteroids even when the body needed them urgently. On top of all this, it must be made very clear that the constant circulation of excessive levels of adrenal hormones of any type can have very damaging implications to health in other ways.

We *do* need sugar to live, but our body is able to take what it needs *slowly and steadily* from the intake of what are known as *complex carbohydrates* (starches), such as:

- Whole grains (such as *brown* rice, whole wheat, oats)
- Beans
- Potatoes (although these are perhaps best avoided

due to the fact that they are a member of the night-shade family – this will be discussed shortly)

What you really want to steer clear from is the *refined sugars* such as white table sugar and brown sugar – even honey should not be used too often.

Caffeine, Nicotine and Alcohol

The major problem with excessive sugar consumption also applies to caffeine, nicotine and alcohol. All three of these cause the indiscriminate release of adrenaline, thus weakening the adrenals and wasting their hormonal supply. The sources of nicotine and alcohol need no introduction, but the more common intake of caffeine can come from several sources, such as:

- Tea
- Coffee
- Chocolate
- Caffeinated soft drinks such as colas
- Certain pain-relieving medications

All three categories make for other problems as well. For instance, aside from the effect on the adrenals, caffeinated coffee and tea appear to be contributing factors in arthritic problems, in part because they drain certain vitamins and minerals from the body which are important in protecting against arthritis.

Tobacco smoking has well-known hazards – many of which are caused by the destructive effect of the smoke-related free radicals that damage tissues in the body and interfere with normal cellular processes. The destruction of tissues is of particular importance here, because collagen matrix is included in the list of victims. Actually, tobacco is a member of the nightshade family of plants, and as such would be restricted even if it were not being smoked! (More about this later.)

Alcohol, besides its negative effects on the adrenal glands, will compromise the joint tissues by draining certain nutrients needed to protect against arthritis. Alcohol also increases the likelihood of a problem mentioned in Chapter Two. You may remember that certain toxins are made when bacteria break down amino acids in the intestines. These toxins inhibit the production of cartilage. Alcohol increases the likelihood of their absorption into the intestinal tract and reduces the ability of the liver to neutralize them before they do their damage.

For these reasons, and many more, it goes without saying that caffeine, nicotine, alcohol *and* refined sugar should be significantly reduced or eliminated from the diet.

Arthritis and the Nightshades

It is much easier to accept that foods we *expect* to be bad for us *are* bad for us. However, when we find out that there are certain foods which we know to be 'healthy' that may nevertheless have to be restricted, the premise is, well, harder to swallow. There certainly is such a dilemma in arthritis. This dilemma relates to a particular category of plants called the *nightshade* family. This category includes:

- Tomatoes
- Peppers (except black)
- White potatoes
- Aubergines (eggplant)
- Tobacco

Now, with the obvious exception of tobacco, the other foods in this list are actually quite nutritious. So why in the world are these foods considered by many to be problematic in arthritis?

Members of this food family contain certain chemicals (solanum alkaloids) that may adversely affect the joints if consumed over long periods. As often is the case, the interest in this particular issue prompted a research study. This research, published in the early 1980s, took place over a seven-year period and involved more than 5,000 volunteers. The results stated that more than 70 per cent of these people, having eliminated nightshades from their diets, experienced improvement over a period of time in their joint pain and discomfort; an improvement in joint integrity was even noticed in many cases. However, as this experiment/survey was conducted through the post, it obviously could not follow strict and controlled guidelines. Nevertheless, the results were quite impressive and certainly do not contradict the anecdotal experiences of many arthritis patients in general, as well as the opinion of many practitioners.

In spite of the fact that the study does not represent unequivocal proof of the value of eliminating the nightshade family from the diet, its results should not be disregarded, especially considering the size of the volunteer group who participated and the length of the study. Therefore, an earnest attempt to follow this example may well be justifiable, at least for certain arthritis sufferers.

'Eat Your Vegetables'

Your mother was right – as usual. While we have covered some of the more negative aspects of diet on arthritis, there are certainly some foods that may be of great value in actually *helping* arthritis sufferers. We have already discussed the benefits of fatty fish. The benefits of fresh vegetables definitely deserve a mention as well.

Free radicals circulate through the body getting in the way and interfering with necessary cellular processes. In arthritis, the end result of this can be significant damage to the joint tissues. It is quite clear from existing research that free radicals are among the most destructive of all influences on the joints.

What is needed is something to neutralize the rampaging free radicals so that the joint tissue cells can carry on as they are supposed to. There is a special name for substances that neutralize free radicals in this way: they are called *antioxidants*.

As you know, our diet can be a major source of free radicals: conversely, our diet can also be a major source of antioxidants! Certain foods contain high amounts of various nutrients that serve as free radical-neutralizers. Some of the main nutrients include:

- Vitamin A
- Beta carotene
- Vitamin C
- Vitamin E
- Selenium (a trace mineral)
- Zinc (a trace mineral)

Some of the richest food sources of these nutrients are:

- Fresh vegetables
- Fresh fruit (remember that it may be advisable to avoid tomatoes and peppers)
- whole grains (*brown* rice, wheat, oats, etc.)
- Beans

All of the foods listed here are not only very good sources of antioxidant vitamins and minerals: they are also excellent sources of *dietary fibre*, which may assist in the removal of toxins in the bowel which exacerbate arthritis in some sufferers. An anti-arthritis diet should probably consist primarily of these foods, as well perhaps as fatty fish such as those listed earlier. A more comprehensive explanation of antioxidants will appear in Part Two of this chapter.

There are certain foods other than the ones listed above that may aggravate arthritis in certain individuals; those mentioned here are only the most common culprits. Keep in mind, too, that an allergy to certain food(s) appears to trigger arthritis symptoms in some sufferers. In such cases it is important for the offending foods to be identified and, if necessary, avoided or eaten only occasionally.

(For more information on food allergies and their treatment, it is suggested you consult the book *Allergies* in this same series.)

PART 2: NUTRITIONAL SUPPLEMENTATION AND HERBAL THERAPY

There certainly is evidence to support the benefits of a healthy diet on arthritis treatment and prevention. These benefits may vary greatly from person to person, but it is important to be patient because sometimes they may take some time to manifest.

What has been particularly exciting on the research front is the *huge* body of evidence that confirms both the therapeutic and preventative benefits of many nutritional substances and herbs. Much of the research also shows that great value can be obtained from such natural agents *without* the risk of side-effects or toxicity seen in orthodox medicines.

The data shows that several vitamins, minerals, amino acids, enzymes, fatty acids and herbs have proven beneficial effects in, among other things:

a Treating the symptoms of arthritis
b Preventing or slowing the development of factors known to cause arthritic damage (such as free radical damage, auto-immunity, lysosomal enzyme damage, etc.)
c Augmenting joint repair

This information has been published over the last several years in the most respected and well-known medical and scientific journals such as *The Lancet, The Journal of the American Medical Association (JAMA)*, the *British Medical Journal*, and the *Journal of Rheumatology*. With this in mind, it is hard to imagine how such information could be relatively unknown to arthritis sufferers. Hopefully, if doctors become more aware of the

proven benefits and high degree of safety of the following natural therapies (as has been shown in their own
professional journals), their patients will be informed
about them as well. After all, a sufferer of *any* disorder
deserves to have easy access to any information that has
been proven to benefit his or her condition. You need
wait no longer, as the next section of this book is dedi-
cated entirely to discussing this information.

Treating Osteoarthritis

ANTIOXIDANTS

One of the main areas of medical and scientific research
over recent years has been the role played by antioxidant therapy in treating and preventing various disorders. The main antioxidant nutrients include:

- Selenium
- Vitamin E
- Zinc
- Vitamin C
- Vitamin A
- Beta carotene

All of these, as well as certain other dietary antioxidants, may play a beneficial role in the treatment
and prevention of arthritic damage. As you know,
antioxidants are the class of substances that are known
to neutralize free radicals. How do they do this? Well,
free radicals circulate through the body with what is
known as an unpaired electron, which basically means
that their molecular structure is partially unattached –
'looking for a dancing partner', if you will. It is in the
nature of free radicals to find something to pair with,

and they do so very effectively. This all sounds very friendly, doesn't it? Well, don't believe it for a minute! The normal and necessary substances in your body have a certain molecular structure that is intended to be the way it is. Any change in that structure causes damage to the substance and, ultimately, to the cells of the tissues affected. When a free radical attaches itself to the structure of a necessary substance, the substance loses its intended characteristics and becomes damaged (and, itself, damaging). This starts a chain reaction which can spread like wildfire.

This is the scenario when free radical damage causes arthritic development in a joint. As you know, superoxides and peroxides cause the most free radical damage in arthritis. As a result, the goal would be to neutralize *these* radicals in particular. There are two main antioxidant enzymes in the body that can carry out this task. They are called *superoxide dismutase (SOD)* and *glutathione peroxidase*. They neutralize superoxide radicals and peroxide radicals, respectively. The antioxidant nutrients selenium and vitamin E help them in their work.

SELENIUM AND VITAMIN E

The antioxidant mineral *selenium* is an essential component of the enzyme glutathione peroxidase in the body. It is needed to elevate the levels of this enzyme so that it can adequately compensate for the damage caused by peroxides. Because of this, selenium is of considerable value in inhibiting joint destruction in osteoarthritis. Selenium-induced glutathione peroxidase also reduces the activity of leukotrienes and inflammatory prostaglandins. Unfortunately, research has shown that selenium levels are significantly depleted in the soil of many parts of Britain and the United States. Naturally, if the soil is depleted of selenium, then people eating foods grown in that soil are likely be deficient in this mineral as well. This is just an observation, but perhaps this is one of the reasons why degenerative arthritis is so prevalent in many Britons and Americans.

Vitamin E is a very well-known vitamin, but not usually with regard to its effects on arthritis. It is very beneficial in the treatment and prevention of osteoarthritis for a few main reasons:

- It increases the activity of selenium
- It enhances the production of cartilage
- It reduces the destruction of joint tissue by lysosomal enzymes
- As an antioxidant it protects against the peroxidation of fats, thereby reducing peroxide damage
- It is an inhibitor of inflammatory prostaglandins

The effects of vitamin E have led to impressive results in clinical research on arthritis patients. Used on its own against a placebo, it was found to have a beneficial effect on osteoarthritic pain. Vitamin E has also been used in arthritis studies in tandem with selenium with very good results. Considering their individual effects, this may come as no surprise, but these two nutrients are synergistic as well. This means that, when used together, the individual effects of each are enhanced. Good news for arthritis sufferers!

ZINC, COPPER AND MANGANESE

These three minerals are particularly important in that they are involved in the production of superoxide dismutase (SOD), which reduces the damage caused by superoxides. Zinc and copper are useful in another way as well, in that they are needed for proper cartilage synthesis.

Injectable SOD, itself, has been used clinically with very positive results. Strangely enough, however, due to its molecular size and structure, oral use of SOD itself would likely be far less effective than injections. Taking zinc, copper and manganese to induce SOD production within the body may well be the preferable method of elevating SOD levels.

VITAMIN C

Vitamin C, perhaps the best-known vitamin, is among the most important nutrients in the fight against osteoarthritis for a few different reasons. First of all, it is the main nutrient needed to make collagen. Since collagen is the most abundant substance in cartilage, and collagen matrix is so heavily destroyed in osteoarthritis, the importance of vitamin C cannot be overstated. The benefit of vitamin C on the maintenance of cartilage is well established in published research. The activity of vitamin C is protective as well due to the fact that it is also a first-class antioxidant nutrient.

Vitamin C has another value as well. It helps to detoxify histamine from the body more quickly. Since histamine is a primary inflammatory chemical, and because it initiates some very tissue-damaging processes, anything that can help to reduce its negative effects is important.

Due to its effect on histamine, its potent free radical-scavenging activity, and its ability to enhance the building of joint tissue, vitamin C should be one of the first considerations in any proposed osteoarthritis programme.

QUERCETIN

In spite of the fact that inflammation is not as prominent in osteoarthritis, the use of anti-inflammatory agents can still play a role in treating its symptoms. Of course in *any* arthritic disorder there are far more factors to treat than just the inflammation. One natural substance that serves a multiple purpose in arthritis treatment is called *quercetin*. Quercetin is classified as a *flavonoid*, that is, part of a family of plant-derived pigmenting agents. It can be found in certain foods (such as onions, broccoli and red cherries), but for therapeutic use it is normally extracted from a herb called *sophora japonicas*. Quercetin is among the most biologically active of all flavonoids. It has a great impact on any form of arthritis for many reasons, including the following:

- It is a very potent inhibitor of inflammation
- It has antioxidant effects
- It has a strengthening effect on collagen matrix
- It reduces the destruction of collagen matrix caused by inflammation-induced lysosomal enzymes

The anti-inflammatory activity of quercetin is well documented in research and is a result of its ability to prevent the body's mast cells from releasing inflammatory agents such as leukotrienes and histamine, as well as its capacity to block production of inflammatory prostaglandins. Even though an anti-inflammatory effect is one of quercetin's main features, as inflammation is less prominent in osteoarthritis the other attributes of this amazing substance may be more important in most cases. Quercetin works extremely well in tandem with vitamin C, both against inflammation and for collagen matrix protection and rebuilding. These two agents deserve a high priority in any arthritis programme.

DL-PHENYLALANINE (DLPA)

Many sufferers would say that it is all very well knowing how to inhibit the development of osteoarthritis; they also would like to know what they can do about the immediate symptoms as well. There is nothing wrong with doing what you can to inhibit the pain and inflammation of arthritis – provided, of course, that doing so does not cause undue damage to the body. We have already looked at the unfortunate implications of using the NSAID class of pain relievers regularly. Not only do you risk the well-known side-effects such as ulcer risk, tinnitus, etc. but there is also the shocking discovery that they *encourage* damage to cartilage.

Fortunately, agents such as quercetin and others help with the inflammation. But what about the chronic pain? Well, as you know, if the inflammation is reduced much of the pain may be diminished as well, due to the fact that chemicals such as histamine stimulate pain fibres. Of course, there is usually far less actual inflammation in osteoarthritis, therefore a significant amount of the pain is likely to be caused by nerve irritation brought on by the deformity, grinding of the joint ends and so on.

Our bodies produce substances called *endorphins* which are chemicals that act to dampen the perception of pain. These are actually morphine-like chemicals, which should give you some idea of the workings of the drug morphine on injured soldiers during the First World War. Another effect of endorphins is that they enhance a person's mood.

The amino acid *DL-phenylalanine (DLPA)* appears to allow a sufferer to maintain higher endorphin levels, thereby reducing his or her perception of pain. Even better news is the fact that DLPA does this without the horrendous addictiveness, toxicity and high risk of side-effects of drugs like morphine.

DLPA is a very safe substance. It is an amino acid made up of L-phenylalanine, a natural amino acid derived from protein, and D-phenylalanine, which is actually a molecular 'mirror image' of the L form. DLPA is a perfect example of how body processes can be stimulated or suppressed without having to use potent drugs. For best results, it is generally recommended that DLPA is taken on an empty stomach. If you suffer from high blood pressure, it should be used only with the consent of the doctor, and only if blood pressure is regularly being monitored.

GLYCOSAMINOGLYCANS

When we look at the matrix of the joint tissue, we see that collagen is a primary constituent. There are other substances involved in the joint connective tissue as well. These are called *glycosaminoglycans* and act as a sort of glue between the cells. As a result of the large amounts of glycosaminoglycans in the connective tissue, it goes without saying that every effort should be made to ensure their protection and production.

There have been efforts to use glycosaminoglycans from animal sources in order to repair damage to human cartilage. Clinical experiments using cattle-derived tracheal cartilage have achieved substantial success. In one such study, only one out of 28 patients did not receive benefits from the administration of the animal cartilage. This sounds remarkably encouraging, but unfortunately these very successful studies involved injection rather than oral administration. Due to the rather large size of the molecules of animal-derived glycosaminoglycans, oral use is not likely to result in intestinal absorption rates high enough to produce similar benefits, although this does not rule out the chance of at least some positive effect. (This, by the way, is also one of the main problems associated with oral administration of SOD.) An extract from green-lipped mussels containing high levels of glycosaminoglycans was found to provide some relief in just over one-third of the patients tested.

L-METHIONINE

Remember, the intestinal barrier is intended to keep out large molecules in the first place. As a result of this protective device, it is vital to try to increase levels of glycosaminoglycans by ingesting their components rather than to hope that the whole molecule is absorbed intact.

One nutrient that is of particular importance in the *production* of glycosaminoglycans is the amino acid *l-methionine*. Methionine is an essential amino acid and as such it is necessary for life. The body cannot make it, however, and thus needs a constant supply from the diet. Methionine contains sulphur, which in itself has been found to be very useful in arthritis treatment. The effects of methionine in glycosaminoglycans production would likely be enhanced by vitamin C, because vitamin C stimulates the growth of a related joint substance called *proteoglycans*.

Remarkably, supplementing l-methionine (in the form of S-adenosyl-methionine) has been found to provide substantial relief in clinical studies. As a matter of fact, it has been suggested in one study that the benefits even exceed those of the popular NSAID, ibuprofen.

DEVIL'S CLAW

The herb devil's claw is, without question, one of the more popular remedies for arthritis in general. The use of this herb has stimulated studies analysing its purported effects. In many of the tests, devil's claw was found to eliminate uric acid from the joints and was described as a strong anti-inflammatory agent and pain reliever. The results of these tests, which were performed on animals, conflicted with the results of other tests, however. While some of the studies showed substantial pain-relieving and anti-inflammatory effects, others did not confirm the substantial anti-inflammatory effect. At this point it would appear that, in spite of the conflicting results, devil's claw is probably well worth trying; keep in mind that benefits may take a matter of weeks to manifest.

YUCCA

Another herb that shows great promise in the treatment of osteoarthritis is *yucca*. Yucca has had a long history of use in the treatment of arthritic conditions. In 1975, a double-blind placebo-controlled clinical study was performed on both osteoarthritis and rheumatoid arthritis patients (most of the patients – just under 60 per cent – had osteoarthritis). The patients were given either yucca saponin extract or a placebo. Over a time period of days, and in some patients more than a few months, over 60 per cent of the yucca-treated patients reported reduced pain, local swelling and joint stiffness.

The reason for these benefits was not completely elucidated, but it is thought that the effect of yucca in arthritis may be due to its effect on toxins produced by bacteria in the intestines. As you may remember, certain bacterial-derived toxins that are absorbed through the intestines can substantially reduce cartilage production.

CONCLUSION

The natural agents that have been discussed are those that may be of greatest use in the treatment and/or prevention of osteoarthritis. It would also be a good idea to insure against any deficiency in nutrients such as the B vitamins, pantothenic acid (vitamin B_5) and niacinamide (vitamin B_3). A deficiency in pantothenic acid is linked to osteoarthritis. Niacinamide has been very successful in clinical studies in treating osteoarthritic symptoms. Unfortunately, the levels of this nutrient that may be needed are quite high, and should only be used on a regular basis at such levels under a doctor's supervision. A multiple vitamin/mineral might be advisable in order to elevate the intake of many nutrients such as these. Even though this might not provide the therapeutic levels needed for nutrients such as niacinamide, at least it may be of benefit to your general state of nutritional health. The list beginning on page 122 outlines a hypothetical supplement programme for osteoarthritis.

Treating Rheumatoid Arthritis

It is clear that there is a great deal of help available for the treatment of osteoarthritis using natural and very safe remedies. The same is most certainly true for rheumatoid arthritis. As you might expect, there are some similarities in the way in which both conditions can be treated, but there are also major differences –

reflecting the two conditions' different causes and slightly different symptoms. In osteoarthritis, a major priority is to lessen the damaging effects of wear and tear as well as free radical-induced joint damage. In the case of rheumatoid arthritis, while these approaches would be helpful, special emphasis really must be put on tackling the severe inflammation and, of course, the damage created by auto-immunity.

FATTY ACIDS (EPA AND GLA)

The role of inflammatory prostaglandins in causing swelling, pain and fever is very well documented. The following is a list of the best ways to reduce the effects of inflammatory prostaglandins such as PGE2:

a Avoid the intake of foods containing the precursor to PGE2 – arachidonic acid.
b Increase the intake of foods that increase the levels of the *anti*-inflammatory prostaglandins. (Earlier in this section you learned that there are also natural substances – such as quercetin – that actually act directly on the cells that produce the inflammatory effect, the mast cells.)
c Increase the intake of substances that inhibit the release of inflammatory chemicals (leukotrienes, hist-amine) and inhibit the production of inflammatory prostaglandins.

In Part One it was mentioned that there are three classes of prostaglandins relevant in arthritis: PG1 series, PG2 series and PG3 series. The body is actually some-what limited as to the amount of prostaglandins that will be produced at a given time. As a result, the greater the intake of the fatty acids required to make a prostaglandin, the greater the likelihood that the effects of that prostaglandin will be pronounced.

In other words, the more arachidonic acid you consume, the more PGE2 will be produced in proportion to the PG1 and 3 series: thus the greater likelihood of inflammatory mechanisms being stimulated. The opposite is also true: the more either PG1 or PG3 or both are produced in the body, the less PG2 series will be produced. This should give you a clue as to the way to proceed. Consume more PG1 and PG3 precursors and less PG2 precursors.

As you know, the precursor of PG2 series is the fatty acid arachidonic acid. This fatty acid is found in animal sources:

• Beef
• Pork
• Lamb
• Dairy products

A precursor of the PG1 series is *gamma linolenic acid (GLA)*. GLA is classed as an *omega 6 fatty acid*. It is found in:

• Evening primrose oil
• Borage seed oil
• Black currant seed oil

Eicosapentaenoic acid (EPA) is a precursor of PG3 series. It is also known as an *omega 3 fatty acid*. Its best natural sources are:

• Salmon
• Mackerel

- Herring
- Cod
- Various other fatty fish

Because these fish are generally cooked before being eaten, it must be remembered that excessive heat denatures unsaturated fats. As a result, it is best that such fish be poached or steamed. Both PG3 precursors can also be obtained in linseed (flaxseed) oil.

There is a growing interest in supplementing the types of oils that increase production of PG1 and PG3 series prostaglandins. No wonder, as there is a substantial body of medical and scientific proof that shows that both EPA and GLA supplements effectively treat arthritis symptoms.

Clinical trials which tested fish oils have shown that *EPA* (which can be found in capsule form) appears to have a measurable anti-inflammatory effect. In the studies, this was manifested by a significant reduction in symptoms, especially pain and stiffness.

The use of *evening primrose oil* has been very impressive as well, showing substantial reduction of symptoms. Interestingly, although it appears that evening primrose does not enhance the relief of symptoms when larger amounts of NSAIDs are used, it does seem to allow the drugs to be reduced in dosage after one to three months. Strangely enough, evening primrose oil, while it works wonders for many sufferers, makes some people seem to get worse for the first week or two. Stranger still, these same sufferers often have been found to benefit the most from evening primrose oil over the long term!

One of the most fascinating facts about evening primrose oil is that it appears either to retard or in some cases, even halt the course of rheumatoid arthritis. This may be due at least in part to the fact that PGE1 helps regulate and restore proper T-cell functioning. This may mean a reduction in or correction of auto-immune tendencies. This would seem to suggest that there is probably a significant imbalance in the body's fatty acids in the first place when rheumatoid arthritis starts to develop. PGE1 also inhibits inflammation-induced lysosomal enzyme damage.

Sources of both EPA and GLA may reduce inflammatory symptoms and subsequent damage by, at least in part, blocking production of prostaglandin E2. Supplements containing these fatty acids should be among the main priorities in any anti-rheumatoid arthritis programme.

QUERCETIN

Quercetin is classified as a *flavonoid*, that is, a plant-derived pigmenting agent. Although it can be found in foods such as onions, broccoli and red cherries, therapeutic amounts would normally be obtained from extracts of quercetin found in a herb called *sophora japonicas*. Quercetin is among the most biologically active of all flavonoids. Although it can have beneficial applications in all forms of arthritis, it should have a particularly profound impact on rheumatoid arthritis at least from a symptomatic standpoint. In the section on osteoarthritis, we looked into its effect on protecting and enhancing collagen matrix. In rheumatoid arthritis this would be the case as well, but the anti-inflammatory effects of quercetin would be especially important. Among quercetin's therapeutic actions are:

- It is a very potent inhibitor of inflammation
- It has antioxidant effects
- It has a strengthening effect on collagen matrix
- It reduces the destruction of collagen matrix due to lysosomal enzymes
- Its anti-inflammatory effect has been well researched. It prevents the release of inflammatory agents such as leukotrienes and histamine from mast cells, as well as blocking production of inflammatory prostaglandins

ANTIOXIDANTS

Over the last several years, but especially recently, medical and scientific research on dietary antioxidants has found them to be among the most important substances in the treatment and prevention of many health disorders. The main antioxidant nutrients include:

- Selenium
- Vitamin E
- Zinc
- Vitamin C
- Beta carotene
- Vitamin A

As mentioned earlier, these nutrients as well as certain other dietary antioxidants may be especially vital in the treatment and prevention of arthritic damage. As the substances that neutralize free radicals, antioxidants protect joint tissue from potent destructive agents. Free radicals circulate through the body with what is known as an unpaired electron. They then spend all of their time trying to attach this electron to something. When they succeed, they proceed to alter the molecular structure of the cellular compound to which they are attached. This change interrupts normal cell processes and thus causes the affected cells to become damaged. This process can start a chain reaction that can spread to other cells if not quelled.

When this occurs in a joint, the resultant damage to the protective tissue cells causes arthritic development. As you know, superoxides and peroxides cause the most free radical damage in arthritis. As a result, it is a major priority to neutralize these radicals in particular. There are two main antioxidant enzymes in the body that function to scavenge these types of free radicals. They are *superoxide dismutase (SOD)* and *glutathione peroxidase*. They neutralize superoxide radicals and peroxide radicals, respectively.

SELENIUM AND VITAMIN E

The antioxidant mineral *selenium* is an essential component of the enzyme glutathione peroxidase. Because of this, selenium intake must be high enough to produce adequate levels of glutathione peroxidase to compensate for the damage caused by peroxides. Selenium is of great value in helping to prevent joint destruction in either rheumatoid or osteoarthritis. To add to that, selenium-induced glutathione peroxidase reduces the activity of inflammatory leukotrienes and prostaglandins. Unfortunately, due to the depleted levels of selenium in the soil of many parts of Britain and the United States, the risks of selenium deficiency are especially high. This may be a major factor in the high prevalence of degenerative arthritis in Britain and the US.

Vitamin E is a well-known fat-soluble vitamin with a potent antioxidant activity. It is highly valuable in the treatment and prevention of rheumatoid arthritis, for the following reasons:

- It increases the activity of selenium
- It enhances the production of cartilage
- It reduces the destruction of joint tissue by lysosomal enzymes
- As an antioxidant, it protects against the peroxidation of fats, thereby reducing peroxide damage
- It is an inhibitor of inflammatory prostaglandins

These benefits help to explain the very successful results received by arthritis patients who participated in clinical trials of vitamin E supplementation. Vitamin E taken on its own was found to reduce the pain of osteoarthritis; in cases of rheumatoid arthritis it was used in tandem with selenium with impressive results. Selenium and vitamin E are synergistic nutrients. This means that when used together, the individual effects of each are enhanced.

ZINC, COPPER AND MANGANESE

The minerals zinc, copper and manganese allow the body to manufacture the other half of the antioxidant enzyme duo, superoxide dismutase (SOD) – which, as you know, reduces the damage of superoxides. Zinc and copper are also required for proper cartilage synthesis.

Injectable SOD, itself, has been very successful in clinical studies. Strangely enough, however, due to its molecular size and structure, oral use of SOD itself would likely be far less effective than injections. Taking zinc, copper and manganese to induce SOD production within the body may well be the preferable method of elevating SOD levels in the body.

VITAMIN C

Vitamin C is among the most important nutrients for arthritis treatment and prevention, for several reasons. First, it is the primary nutrient needed to make collagen, the most abundant substance in cartilage. As collagen matrix is destroyed in degenerative arthritis, the importance of vitamin C is clear. The benefits of vitamin C on cartilage are validated in published research. Not only does vitamin C play a vital role in the production of cartilage, it also helps maintain bone matrix as well.

As a primary antioxidant, vitamin C is an effective inhibitor of free radical damage and retards potentially joint-damaging substances. It also helps to detoxify histamine in the body more quickly. Histamine is, as you know, a potent inflammatory chemical and as such can eventually initiate joint-damaging processes. As a result, histamine detoxification is certainly an important asset where rheumatoid arthritis is concerned.

SCUTELLARIA BAICALENSIS

The Chinese herb *scutellaria baicalensis* has been the subject of very important and impressive research which confirms that it has a potent anti-inflammatory and anti-arthritic effect. It has been suggested that the activity of the naturally occurring flavonoids contained in scutellaria compare quite favourably to certain commonly prescribed NSAIDs, without their common side-effects.

Scutellaria also possesses a significant anti-allergic effect and has the ability to block production of very potent inflammatory substances such as leukotrienes. This anti-allergic effect would have some relevance in rheumatoid arthritis, as inflammatory mechanisms appear to be allergy-induced in some or perhaps many sufferers. Although this herb is less well known to date than some of the other anti-arthritic agents, it has held up well to scientific and medical scrutiny and may be one of the most promising remedies of all.

DL-PHENYLALANINE (DLPA)

To many rheumatoid arthritis sufferers, the reduction of pain may be an even more important priority than treating the cause of the disease's development. While this may not be the most effective way to approach the problem, it is nevertheless only right that sufferers have adequate relief from the worst symptoms. As the negative effects of NSAID pain-relievers are brought to light, the need to have a safer alternative – especially one that does not actually *worsen* joint degeneration – becomes more obvious. Agents such as quercetin and scutellaria may help with the inflammation; if the inflammation is reduced, much of the pain may be reduced. As rheumatoid arthritis advances, however, at least some of the pain is likely to be generated by nerve irritation caused by deformity of the bones and the grinding of the joint ends.

Our bodies produce natural pain-killing chemicals called *endorphins*. These chemicals dampen the body's perception of pain. Morphine-like, these chemicals not only hinder pain perception, but also function to elevate a person's mood.

It appears that the amino acid *DL-phenylalanine (DLPA)* allows sufferers to maintain higher endorphin levels, thereby reducing their perception of pain. DLPA seems to accomplish this without the severe addictiveness, toxicity and high risk of side-effects of drugs such as morphine.

DLPA is made up of L-phenylalanine, a natural amino acid derived from protein, and D-phenylalanine, which is a molecular 'mirror image' of the L form. As previously mentioned, for best results, it is generally recommended that DLPA is taken on an empty stomach. If you suffer from high blood pressure, it should be used only with the consent of the doctor, and only if blood pressure is regularly being monitored.

DEVIL'S CLAW

One of the more common natural remedies for the treatment of arthritis is the herb devil's claw. In some experimental studies on animals, devil's claw was reported to eliminate uric acid from the joints and to be a strong anti-inflammatory agent and pain reliever. Other tests suggested that it was not such an effective anti-inflammatory agent. In spite of these conflicting results, devil's claw is probably worth a try – keep in mind that it may take several weeks before there is any noticeable improvement in your symptoms.

BROMELAIN

Another potent agent with research-proven anti-inflammatory effects is an enzyme derived from pineapple called *bromelain*.

Bromelain has generated a great deal of interest because of its proven ability to dissolve atherosclerotic blood clots. Its ability to reduce inflammation very quickly is also worth noting. One of the particularly important effects of bromelain in rheumatoid arthritis, besides its ability to reduce inflammation, is that it can help to remove antibody complexes which can injure joint tissue.

As bromelain is a strong protein-digesting enzyme it is suggested that, if being taken for inflammation, it should be taken on an empty stomach so that it can be most active working on inflammatory agents rather than food.

DIGESTIVE ENZYMES

In spite of the fact that a digestive aid such as bromelain will ordinarily be used as an anti-inflammatory in arthritis treatment, there is a very good case to be made for the use of digestive aids *after* meals as well. It is important to remember that food allergens (antigens) can cause an inflammatory effect in a joint and/or cause a hyperactivity of antibodies that may inadvertently cross-react with joint tissue. When you consider this, it becomes all the more clear that it is important to do everything in your power to eliminate food allergens in the first place.

The substances that are most likely to produce an allergic reaction are: incompletely digested proteins and, less frequently, carbohydrates. The truth is, if the proteins or carbohydrates contained in a particular food are completely digested in the first place, then they are theoretically not capable of causing an allergy.

It would appear that poor digestion may be a major factor in many cases of rheumatoid arthritis. This would certainly be the case in those whose arthritis is exacerbated by a food allergy or allergies. In these individuals it may be recommended that they enhance the digestion of proteins and carbohydrates by using *betaine hydrochloride* and *pancreatic enzymes*.

Betaine hydrochloride is a supplemental form of the enzyme hydrochloric acid (which the body releases into the stomach to digest proteins). Many people have exceedingly low levels of this enzyme and thus may benefit by its supplementation. Betaine hydrochloride must only be taken during or immediately after meals; it should *not* be taken if you suffer with a stomach or duodenal ulcer – in these cases check first with your doctor.

Pancreatin contains the enzymes that are produced by the pancreas and released into the duodenum (the first part of the small intestine). Pancreatic enzymes such as protease, amylase and lipase digest proteins, carbohydrates and fats respectively.

Supplementing betaine hydrochloride and pancreatic enzymes may reduce significantly the risk of the body absorbing incompletely digested food components into the bloodstream.

(For more information on food allergies and their treatment, it is suggested you consult the book *Allergies* in this same series.)

CONCLUSION

The supplements mentioned in this section may be very useful in treating the symptoms as well as various factors involved in the development of rheumatoid arthritis. It may also be a good idea to make sure you are getting enough of all the essential nutrients your body needs, perhaps by taking multiple vitamin and multiple mineral supplements. The list below outlines a hypothetical supplement programme for rheumatoid arthritis, as well as a basic recommendation for the other forms of arthritis discussed in this book.

PLEASE NOTE: The following information is *not* intended to be prescriptive. The author and the publisher accept no responsibility for any circumstances that result from the reader experimenting with the following programmes. Please consult a doctor before beginning this or any other new health regime.

OSTEOARTHRITIS
Avoid or reduce the intake of:

- Fried foods and oils cooked at very high temperatures hydrogenated fats
- Dairy products (unless non-fat or very low fat – none if you are allergic to them)
- Alcohol
- Tobacco
- Caffeine
- Refined sugar
- Red meat
- Tomatoes
- Peppers (except black)
- Aubergines (eggplant)
- Potatoes

Hypothetical recommendations (adult dosages):

- Antioxidants (and antioxidant enzyme-inducers) [many are available in antioxidant combinations]:
  ° Vitamin A and/or beta carotene (7,500–15,000 IU, once daily)
  ° Vitamin C (500–1,000 mg, 2–3 times daily)
  ° Vitamin E (200–400 IU, 1–2 times daily)
  ° Selenium (100–200 mcg, once daily)
  ° Zinc – picolinate or amino acid chelate (20–25 mg, once daily)
  ° Copper – amino acid chelate (1–2 mg, once daily)
  ° Manganese – amino acid chelate (5–15 mg, once daily)
- Quercetin (250–500 mg, twice daily between meals)
- DL-phenylalanine (DLPA) (300–500 mg, 2–3 times daily taken on an empty stomach – if you have high

blood pressure, take with food and only on the advice of your doctor)

- L-methionine: (400–500 mg, twice daily on an empty stomach. When taking methionine as a supplement, make sure your vitamin B_6 intake is adequate, for example by taking a multiple vitamin or B-complex supplement)
- Devil's claw: (500–1,000 mg, twice daily)
- Yucca (1,000–1,500 mg, twice daily)
- Multiple vitamin/mineral (with minimum 40–50 mg B-complex, as directed)

RHEUMATOID ARTHRITIS

Avoid or reduce the intake of:

- Fried foods and oils cooked at very high temperatures
- Hydrogenated fats
- Dairy products (unless non-fat or very low fat – none if you are allergic to them)
- Alcohol
- Tobacco
- Caffeine
- Refined sugar
- Red meat
- Tomatoes
- Peppers (except black)
- Aubergines (eggplant)
- Potatoes
- Any foods you are allergic to

Hypothetical recommendations (adult dosages)

- EPA (300–800 mg, 2–3 times daily)
  (Do not take if using prescription anticoagulants such

as warfarin, except with the consent of your doctor)

- GLA – as evening primrose oil or borage oil (50–100 mg, 2–3 times daily)
- Quercetin (250–500 mg, twice daily between meals)
- Antioxidants (and antioxidant enzyme inducers) [many are available in antioxidant combinations]:
  - ° Vitamin A and/or beta carotene (7,500–15,000 IU once daily)
  - ° Vitamin C (500–1,000 mg, 2–3 times daily)
  - ° Vitamin E (200–400 IU, 1–2 times daily)
  - ° Selenium (100–200 mcg, once daily)
  - ° Zinc – picolinate or amino acid chelate (20–25 mg, once daily)
  - ° Copper – amino acid chelate (1–2 mg, once daily)
  - ° Manganese – amino acid chelate (5–15 mg, once daily)
- Scutellaria baicalensis (500–1,000 mg, twice daily)
- DL-phenylalanine (DLPA) (300–500 mg, 2–3 times daily taken on an empty stomach – if you have high blood pressure, take only on the advice of your doctor)
- Bromelain (400–500 mg, 2–3 times daily between meals)
- Devil's claw (500–1,000 mg, twice daily)
- Betaine hydrochloride (300–600 mg, during or immediately after each major protein-containing meal (do *not* take if you have a stomach or duodenal ulcer/reduce dosage if you experience unusual warmth in your stomach after taking it)
- Pancreatin – quadruple strength (500–1,000 mg, during or immediately after each major meal)
- Multiple vitamin/mineral (with minimum 40–50 mg B-complex, as directed)

GENERAL RHEUMATISM AND SPORTS INJURIES

Avoid or reduce the intake of:

- Fried foods and oils cooked at very high temperatures
- Hydrogenated fats
- Dairy products (unless non-fat or very low fat)
- Alcohol
- Tobacco
- Caffeine
- Refined sugar
- Red meat
- Tomatoes
- Peppers (except black)
- Aubergines (eggplant)
- Potatoes

Hypothetical recommendations (adult dosages)

- EPA (300–800 mg, 2–3 times daily)
  (Do *not* take if using prescription anticoagulants such as warfarin, except with the consent of your doctor)
- Quercetin (250–500 mg, twice daily between meals)
- Bromelain: (400–500 mg, 2–3 times daily between meals)
- Antioxidants (the following may be obtainable in antioxidant combinations):
  - Vitamin A and/or beta carotene (7,500–15,000 IU, once daily)
  - Vitamin C (500–1,000 mg, 2–3 times daily)
  - Vitamin E (200–400 IU, 1–2 times daily)
  - Selenium (100–200 mcg, once daily)
  - Zinc – picolinate or amino acid chelate (20–25 mg, once daily)
- Scutellaria baicalensis (500–1,000 mg, twice daily)

CHAPTER 5

Making the Most of
Your Programme

There is little question that a great deal of emotional relief accompanies the realization that there really *is* something that can be done about even the most serious forms of arthritis. Even more encouraging is the fact that this information is not merely the product of anecdotal, historical or theoretical data. It is really quite exciting to see the vast amount of research data being published in medical and scientific journals which shows both the efficacy and safety of natural medicine.

In spite of this, it must be reiterated that you should always let your doctor know if you are considering a new health programme. This will give him or her the opportunity to give advice relative to your particular medical circumstances. Part of this is precautionary, in that, although very unusual, at times there are special contra-indications if you are already on certain medication. Even if you are not on medication, there are also some rare medical circumstances which would suggest an alteration in such a programme. The programmes discussed in the last chapter are only hypothetical in any case, based on current knowledge of the substances that have been found generally to help alleviate the suffering caused by various forms of arthritis; these programmes cannot take into consideration each person's unique biochemistry.

At any rate, before you begin any such programme, make sure that you are certain about the diagnosis of your type of arthritis. Although there are obviously some similarities between the different programmes listed in Chapter Four, the greatest benefits are more likely if you follow a programme specific to your condition. This is especially the case if you are interested in more than just temporarily relieving the symptoms.

It is sometimes advisable to begin with a lower intake per day of the various supplements until you are accustomed to the programme. Once you are sure that you feel comfortable with the supplementation, then normally the intake is increased to the approximate range listed. This is not by any means always necessary, but may be a good idea, particularly if the entire programme is followed. The supplements listed are very safe, especially in the dosages listed, but very rarely a person may need to adjust the programme in the event that he or she does not tolerate a particular substance well. If this should prove the case, simply stop taking the supplement that does not agree with you (trial and error will help pinpoint which supplement this is). Do not be too disappointed should this occur, as there may well be another supplement in the programme which can compensate, at least somewhat, for the benefits of the supplement you have had to eliminate.

As you might expect, many people would rather take a tablet or capsule than follow a restricted diet. This is human nature, but the foods mentioned in Chapter Four as being problematic really can exacerbate arthritis. And while we know from the research that many substances help to combat arthritis even when no special restricted diet is followed, who knows how much more substantial and fast the benefits might be if an 'anti-arthritic' diet is followed at the same time? The wisdom of making dietary changes, such as eliminating certain fats, has been proven in arthritis studies. The elimination of meat from the diet of arthritis sufferers has a proven and noticeable benefit as well. The detrimental effects of tobacco, caffeine, alcohol and sugar are well-documented and are relevant to many different health disorders. There is at least some clinical evidence of the apparent advantage of eliminating the class of nightshade foods. In other words, for the greatest (and quickest) good to come of an arthritis programme, do not neglect the dietary recommendations just because you are reaping the benefits of supplementation.

It is certainly a personal decision as to how strictly you choose to follow either the dietary or supplementation part of the programme, but it helps to be reminded of the attributes of both. In order to avoid any undue stress caused by having to change your daily routine enormously and all at once, find a way of 'phasing in' such changes at a pace that suits you and your lifestyle best. If you are the type of person who makes changes easily, then you can be more bold in your adoption of a programme. If, on the other hand, your life is not conducive to immediate change, use your discretion as to how best to wean yourself onto a new regime. If you 'cheat' on your diet and sneak a pepperoni and sausage pizza, or if you miss a day's supplements for some reason, *do not* think that you have ruined everything – because you haven't – and by all means, *do not* give up. Just get back on track. Getting angry and disappointed with yourself is more likely to *de*-motivate you, so keep a positive attitude regardless of whether or not you have an occasional lapse. Once you have hit your stride and have some experience under your belt, the programme will become much easier to follow.

The information in Chapter Four is by no means the only non-drug method available. In order to increase the benefits of your new programme even further, you can also adopt various external approaches such as hydrotherapy, massage, acupuncture and so on. These areas cannot be covered in detail here, so your best bet may be to speak to a qualified practitioner of one or all of these therapies in order to get an idea of whether they would be of interest to you.

As you can see, there are really *many* different ways to help alleviate both the symptoms and development of arthritis. Of course, prevention is always best, but even when arthritis has set in, it is not too late to try to prevent its further development.

The methods that have been discussed in this book offer great promise and have, of course, already been analysed from a medical and/or scientific standpoint. Now it is up to you to analyse them for yourself. They may well provide you with what you need to gain effective and safe control over your arthritis and end your suffering for good!

BIBLIOGRAPHY

Amella, M. *et al. Planta Medica*, 51, 1985, pp. 16–20.

Bingham, R. *et al. Journal of Applied Nutrition*, 27, 1975, pp. 45–50.

Bland, J. & Cooper, S. *Seminars in Arthritis and Rheumatism*, 14, 1984, pp. 106–33.

Brady, L. *et al. Pharmacognosy* (8th ed.), Lea and Febiger, 1981, p. 480.

British Medical Association. *Guide to Medicines and Drugs*, Dorling Kindersley, 1991.

Brook, P. *et al. Journal of Rheumatology*, 9, 1982, pp. 3–5.

Burton, G. & Ingold, K. *Science*, 224, 1984, pp. 569–73.

Childers, N. *Journal of the International Academy of Preventive Medicine*, July 1982, pp.5–16.

Childers, N. & Russo, G. *The Nightshades and Health*, Horticultural Pub., 1973.

Chung i yen chiu yuan chung yao yen chiu ssu (ed.). *Chinese Medical Journal*, 7, 1973, pp. 417–20.

Cirelli, M. *Clinical Medicine*, 74, 6, 1967, pp. 55–9.

Cohen, A. & Goldman, J. *Pennsylvania Medical Journal*, 67, June 1964, pp. 27–30.

Cotzias, G. *et al. Journal of Clinical Investigation*, 47, 1968, p. 992.

Cragin, R. *Medical Times*, 90, 1962, pp. 529–30.

Darlington, L. *et al. The Lancet*, 1 Feb., 1986, pp. 236–8.

Di Padova, C. *American Journal of Medicine*, 83, 1987, pp. 60–65.

Eichler, O. & Koch, C. *Arzneim Forsch*, 20, 1, 1970, p. 107.

Erdos, A. *et al. Planta Medica*, 34, 1978, p. 97.

Ferreira, S. & Nakamura, M. *Prostaglandins*, 18, 1979, pp. 191–200.

Goebel, K. *et al. The Lancet*, 1, 1981, pp. 1,015–17.

Hansen, T. *et al. Scandinavian Journal of Rheumatism*, 12, 1983, p. 85.

Hartz, A. *et al. Journal of Chronic Dis.*, 39, 1986, pp. 311–19.

Havsteen, B. *Biochemical Pharmacology*, 32, 1983, pp. 1,141–8.

Hicklin, J. *et al. Clinical Allergy*, 10, 1980, p. 463.

Horrobin, D. *Journal of Holistic Medicine*, 3, 1981, pp. 118–39.

International Journal of Vitamins and Nutritional Research (suppl.), 26, 1984, pp. 141–6.

Ito, C. *et al. Folia Pharmacol. Japan*, 75, 1979, pp. 227–37.

Kamimura, M. *Journal of Vitaminology*, 18, 1972, pp. 204–9.

Kimura, Y. *et al. Planta Medica*, 54, 1985, pp. 132–6.

Kremer, J. *et al. The Lancet*, 1,

1985, pp. 184–7.

Krupp, M. & Chatton, M. (eds.). *Current Medical Treatment and Diagnosis*, Lange Medical Pub., 1982.

Krystal, G. *et al. Arth. Rheum.*, 25, 1982, pp. 318–25.

Kubo, M. *et al. Chem. Pharm. Bulletin*, 32, 1984, pp. 2,724–9.

Kunkel, S. *et al. Prog. Lipid Research*, 20, 1–4, 1981, pp. 885–8.

Lee, T. *et al. New England Journal of Medicine*, 312, 1985, pp. 1,217–23.

Lewis, A. *Agents and Actions*, 15, 1984, pp. 513–19.

Little, C. *et al. The Lancet*, 2, 1983, p. 297.

Lucas, C. & Power, L. *Clinical Research*, 29, 4, 1981, p. 754a.

Lucas, C & Power, L. *Journal of the American Medical Association*, 9 April, 1982.

Machtey, I & Ouaknin, L. *Journal of the American Geriatrics Society*, 26, 1978, pp. 328–30.

Marcolongo, R. *et al. Current Therapeutic Research*, 37, 1985, pp. 82–94.

Marone, G. *et al. Agents and Actions*, 18, 1986, pp. 103–6.

Meander-Huber, K. *European Journal of Rheumatology and Inflammation*, 4, 1981, p. 62.

Middleton, E. & Drzewieki, G. *Archives of Allergy and Applied Immunology*, 77, 1985, pp. 155–7.

Millinger, G. *Cranio*, 4, 2, 1986, pp. 156–63.

Moore, K. *Clinically Oriented Anatomy* (3rd ed.), Williams & Wilkins, 1992.

Munthe, E. & Aseth, J. *Scandinavian Journal of Rheumatology*, 53 suppl., 1984, p. 103.

Murray, M. & Pizzorno, J. *Encyclopaedia of Natural Medicine*, Macdonald and Co., 1990.

Nandi, B. *et al. Biochemical Pharmacology*, 23, 1974, pp. 643–7.

Nelson, N. *et al. Chemical and Engineering News*, 16 August, 1982, p. 80.

Newman, M. & Ling, R. *The Lancet*, ii, 1985, pgs. 11–13.

Pandley, S. *et al. Indian Journal of Medical Research*, 81, 1985, pp. 618–20.

Parish, P. *Medical Treatments: The Benefits and Risks*, Penguin, 1991.

Pasquier, C. *et al. Inflammation*, 8, 1984, pp. 27–32.

Roberts, P. *et al. Med. Biol.*, 62, 1984, p. 88.

Schauf, C. *et al. Human Physiology*, Times Mirror/Mosby, 1990.

Segal, A. *et al.*, *British Journal of Rheumatology*, 25, 1986, pp. 162–6.

Shahied, I. *Biochemistry of Food and the Biocatalysts*, Vantage, 1977, pp. 171–80, 251–9.

Sorensen, J. *Journal Med. Chem.*, 19, 1976, p. 126.

Spencer, H. and Osis, D. *American Journal of Clinical Nutrition*, 36, 1982, p. 776.

Taraye, J. & Lauessergues, H. *Arzneim-Forsch*, 27, 1, 1977, pp. 1,144–9.

Tarp, U. *et al. Scandinavian Journal of Rheumatology*, 14, 1985, pp. 364–8.

Tarp, U. *et al. Scandinavian Journal of Rheumatology*, 14, 1985, p. 97.

Vacha, J. *et al. Arzneim-Forsch*, 34, 1984, pp. 607–9.

Werbach, M. *Nutritional Influences on Illness*, Thorsons, 1991.

Zaphiropoulos, G. *British Journal of Rheumatology*, 25, 1986, pp. 138–40.

INDEX